C000196371

OESTROGEN
THE KILLER IN OUR MIDST

Third Edition

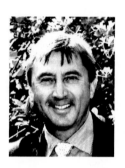

Chris has a degree in biochemistry from Oxford University and has formally studied both cancer and nutrition. He is a founder of the Integrative CANCERactive charity and editor for its 3600 page website and the magazine **icon**, which is provided free to people touched by cancer in over 640 hospitals and cancer centres in the UK. He is a tireless cancer researcher, with several books to his name. He fervently believes that we already know enough to cure cancer or at least hold it in permanent remission, but that we simply do not use the research knowledge that is already available throughout the world. He is much in demand as a speaker and has spoken on multiple occasions in the USA, Russia, Japan and Australia apart from a tour with TV and media appearances all round Britain and Ireland.

OESTROGEN
THE KILLER IN OUR MIDST

Third Edition

How to combat one of the biggest health threats today

Chris Woollams M.A. (Oxon)

Copyright © 2004 by Chris Woollams.

Chris Woollams asserts the moral right to be identified as the author of this work.

A catalogue record for this book is available from the British Library.

All rights reserved. No part of this book may be reproduced or transmitted in any form or by any means, electronic or mechanical, including photocopying, recording, or by any information storage retrieval system, without permission in writing from the publisher and the author.

First published in March 2004 by Health Issues Ltd
Second edition: January 2006
Third edition, now published by CANCERactive, Feb 2014

Cover design by Jeremy Baker.

ISBN 978-0-9565391-4-4

Printed in England by CPI Group (UK) Ltd, Croydon CR04YY.
And printed in Australia by Griffin Press, Adelaide.

Important Notice

This info-book represents a review and an interpretation of a vast number of varied sources available to anyone on the subject of oestrogen and cancer.

Whilst the author has made every effort to ensure that the facts, information and conclusions are accurate and as up to date as possible at the time of publication, the author and publisher assume no responsibility.

The author is neither a fully qualified Health Practitioner nor a Doctor of Medicine and so is not qualified to give any advice on any medical matters. Cancer (and its related illnesses) is a very serious and very individual disease, and readers must consult with experts and specialists in the appropriate medical field before taking, or refraining from taking, any action.

This book and the advice contained are not intended as an alternative to such specialist advice, which should be sought for accurate diagnosis and before any course of treatment.

The author and the publisher cannot be held responsible for any action, or lack of action, that is taken by any reader as a result of information contained in the text of this book. Such action is taken entirely at the reader's own risk.

Nothing so needs reforming
as other peoples' habits.

Mark Twain

CONTENTS

INTRODUCTION

I wanted to write this book for simple reasons: Firstly, women with breast cancer are routinely tested for oestrogen, progesterone and HER-2 links. Some 70 per cent of women will be told that their cancers are driven by oestrogen and typically the treatment will include 5 years of Tamoxifen to block receptor sites from the action of oestrogen, then three years of a drug such as Arimidex which aims to cut oestrogen production around the body. Many women want to take some control over their own lives and their fight against cancer, and they need to be aware that there is a great deal they can do in their general habits and lifestyle that will help their oestrogen reduction programme. This book is for them.

However, there are many, many women who are afraid that they might fall victim to the horrors of breast cancer and so want to take all sensible steps possible to prevent this occurring. This book is for them, too.

But there is clear research that a host of other cancers may also be driven by oestrogen. For example there is research showing the following cancers have links to oestrogen: Brain tumours, prostate cancer, testicular cancer, colon cancer, stomach cancer, lung cancer, ovarian cancer, endometrial cancer and several more. In each case, as with breast cancer, not every cancer is linked to oestrogen, just a proportion. What is apparent from this list is that this is far from a list exclusive to women. Oestrogen, the female sex hormone, drives male cancers too. This book is for all these people, male and female too.

This book will save men and women with hormonally driven cancers a lot of time. It will empower them to make their own contribution to their *Complementary and Integrative* cancer treatment programme.

In some of my other books I cover The American Cancer Society's 2012 report: that since 2006 there has been an 'explosion' in research into complementary therapies and that there is 'overwhelming evidence' that some, such as diet, exercise and weight control, can increase survival and keep you cancer free.

The Block Center for Integrative Medicine in Illinois has conducted clinical research which clearly shows that women who built a Complementary and Integrative cancer treatment programme survived at least twice as long as those who did not.

This book will also save me a lot of time. Hormonally driven cancer is so common I have often had the same conversation five times in just a few hours!

I want to make a couple of final points very clearly. I write for ordinary people touched by cancer, not for scientists, pseudo-scientists or skeptic critics. So I write in an easy-to-understand format, in *peoplespeak* not *sciencespeak*. The action of oestrogen in the body and the genes involved is very complex. The aim wasn't to delve into deep scientific theory; it was to present sufficient knowledge so that people could form a plan of action by making more informed personal choices in their lives.

I am also told by people with cancer that they simply do not want or need the clutter of references. But if you do need a reference just go to one of three places on www.canceractive.com: the research centre Cancer Watch, or the articles in the section Your Cancer – Breast Cancer, or to four articles called The four pillars of cancer. It really is all there.

Finally, I'd like to thank Professor Trevor Powles, the late Dr John Lee, Dr Tessa Pollard, Dr Francisco Contreras, Dr Julian Kenyon, Dr Philippa Darbre, Sherrill Sellman, Professor Karol Sikora, Dr Rosy Daniel, and staff at The Haven in London who all indirectly and inadvertently helped provide me with research and ideas that I have used in this book! Plus of course Lindsey, Maggie, Melanie, Madeleine, Susan, Janet, Jeremy, Wendy, and Jane who read, commented on, and typed . . . and retyped!

Chris Woollams
December 2013

CHAPTER 1

WHAT ARE HORMONES AND WHAT'S THE PROBLEM?

Hormones are super-chemicals - the body's messengers. Even very small amounts of hormones have a monstrous effect on the actions of the human body. One part in a trillion or even quadrillion is all it takes for a hormone chemical to have a major effect.

Conventional theory runs that hormones are produced by your endocrine glands, for example – your pituitary, pineal gland, adrenal glands (kidneys), ovaries, thyroid, testes, etc.

These organs are directly under the command of the brain and the nervous system. This is most obvious when an animal is placed in a state of fear. When sensing danger the brain stimulates the production of adrenalin, the 'fight or flight' hormone, which prepares our whole body for immediate action.

Two facts about hormones are particularly relevant to the cancer issue:

1. Hormones can cause chronic Inflammation

Not all hormones are produced in the endocrine glands. In fact the vast majority of these super-chemicals are not! It is a little known fact **that every single cell in your body has the ability to produce localised hormones.** Back in 1982, John Vane won a knighthood and a Nobel Prize for his work on

1

eicosanoids, hormones that last but a few seconds and are produced by the nuclear envelope in every cell in your body. There are about 130 different eicosanoids, some good, some bad. You may have heard of prostaglandins. If their levels increase they can increase the risk of inflammatory arthritis in your joints. And that is really what excesses of 'bad' eicosanoids do: They increase inflammation at the cellular level.

The implications of this discovery are huge. For example, it is known that cortisol, the 'stress' hormone, can stimulate an enzyme (called COX-2) to produce more 'bad' eicosanoids thus making the environment of that cell inflamed. In simple terms, what this means is: Your brain becomes stressed, it sends a message to your adrenal glands and these produce cortisol and, in turn, your breast cells or prostate cells become stressed too!! Stressed brain, stressed breast. The hormone insulin, produced in response to glucose in the blood stream, also has a similar, effect on COX-2 at this cellular level.

Chronic inflammation at the cellular level lies behind cancer development. And Tian Xu, Professor of Genetics at the *Yale Medical Centre* confirmed *'What other people felt was true, but couldn't prove'*. He showed that emotional stress caused chronic inflammation, which in turn stimulates two cancer-causing genes inside the cell *(Nature, Jan 2010)*.

Cancer research UK has produced research showing that stress in the work place is not linked to increased risks of cancer. But the stress of the loss of a mother or a child, problems of a daughter's marriage or financial situation certainly do cause many women a great deal of emotional stress, which they would argue tipped them over the edge in causing their breast cancer. The above science from Vane and Xu would lend support to that argument.

Furthermore, when people develop cancer their stress hormone levels subsequently increase. This results in more inflammation around the body at a localised level. UCLA and Harvard Medical Schools have conducted a number of research studies on this subject and all are covered in Cancer Watch, the CANCERactive research centre. Suffice it to say here that localised inflammation serves the cancer well as it enables metastases to take charge.

But people with cancer can fight back. One of the best ways of reducing inflammation is through diet; employing a Rainbow Mediterranean Diet comes out a clear winner. Yoga was shown by Seattle Medical School to have a strong ability to reduce cortisol levels, by as much as 25 per cent on your first ever yoga class; 40 per cent by the end of the first week. Whereas following doctor's orders and resting for a week only reduced stress cortisol levels by five per cent. According to research from UCLA Transcendental Meditation beats all of this for reducing cortisol and other stress hormone levels in the body. And a large clinically controlled study showed that people who used Stress Management Courses (all of the above, plus counselling) survived 'significantly longer'.

But that takes care of the cortisol. We can also tackle the insulin.

Obviously, this involves diet since insulin is stimulated by increased levels of plasma glucose. For a start, reduce all consumption of glucose, refined carbohydrates, biscuits, cake, chocolate, fizzy soft drinks and the rest of the junk. Not only does this cause insulin surges, glucose is the favourite food of a cancer cell. It needs lots to survive and grow. Without glucose cancer cells can turn sometimes to glutamine, from protein, but essentially they are in trouble. Healthy cells, on the other hand can just switch over to burning fats if there is insufficient glucose around. It's called ketosis.

Both Calorie Restriction (where people consume roughly 15 per cent less calories than they need), and Fasting for three to five days, have been shown to lower levels of insulin, IGF-1 (growth hormone) and oestrogen in the blood. Both have been associated with halting cancer progression, and the use of such techniques has improved the outcomes in patients having chemo- or radiotherapy too.

At the simplest level, you should graze, eating five or six small meals a day, and avoiding the large 'blow out' meal, especially in the evening.

But what of trying to stop the action of COX-2? Again, this is diet related:

a) Vane argued that a small (75 mg) aspirin would reduce COX-2's action. Since his time there has been more research, notably from the Mayo Clinic (same conclusion but recommending 81 mgs) and

4

Oxford University and the Radcliffe who in 2012 concluded that taking a small daily dose of aspirin would reduce the risk of developing cancer and, if you already had it, would reduce metastases and greatly increase survival times; so much so that they asked NICE to approve daily aspirin as part of all cancer treatment programmes in the UK!

b) Since Vane's research other cancer centres have noted that fish oils, curcumin, resveratrol, garlic and ginger can all reduce COX-2 action. Aloe Vera has a similar benefit in the colon.

Fish oils have several other benefits, one particularly important. Think of your DNA as a shoe lace, having at either end the piece of plastic that holds it together. With DNA the two ends are called telomeres. As you age they shorten. If you have cancer, they shorten dramatically. But fish oil consumption can re-lengthen them, according to UCLA research.

2. Hormone imbalance can stimulate cancer pathways

While chronic inflammation is one pathway to cancer, there are others. And oestrogen and Insulin-like growth hormone (IGF-1) amongst other hormones, can influence such pathways.

In a healthy animal enjoying a totally natural, clean living life, **its hormones are totally in balance within the body.** This is called **homeostasis.**

However, when one single hormone is suddenly heightened or reduced, there is a knock-on effect to all the other hormones throughout the body. Some are increased, others decrease.

In the modern world much of the disruption of the 'normal' hormone balance is caused by our own habits and actions. For example, as we covered above, eating large carbohydrate-rich meals, stimulates huge rises in the hormones insulin and IGF-1. Consuming cows' dairy also heightens IGF-1 levels in the body.

A lack of exercise will affect 'normal' hormone levels too, since exercise has, for example, been shown to produce endorphins which help regulate stress hormones, and exercise helps control plasma glucose levels.

But it doesn't have to be a human hormone causing the disruption. Chemicals from external sources can disrupt your hormone balance; they can be called hormone disrupters or xenoestrogens. You can find them in pesticides. In Israel forty years ago, the pesticides DDT and Lindane were shown to lie behind the extraordinarily high levels of breast cancer; almost four times those of Europe. The pesticides were getting into the food chain via cows grazing contaminated fields and then women drinking their milk. Milk fat is a wonderful solvent for such toxins.

In 2013 The World Health Organisation produced a report asking governments to urgently ban certain common chemicals of concern: For example, BPA (a component of the plastic in many plastic bottles, wrappers, plastic cups, toys and the white lining of cans), **phthalates** (from plasticisers in many bottles) and **parabens** (a common preservative). All are hormone disrupters.

If governments take no action, I'm afraid you need to vote with your wallet.

CHAPTER 2
ARE OTHER HORMONES INVOLVED IN CANCER?

So that briefly covers the involvement of cortisol, eicosanoids, IGF-1 and insulin, while oestrogen we will cover in more detail shortly. A couple of other hormones are worth a mention at this point:

Thyroxine is the hormone of the Thyroid. Women with low thyroid hormone levels develop less cancer, but women with high thyroid hormone levels develop more. The pathway has been identified and is not the same as that stimulated by oestrogen. Importantly, there is some concern for women who supplement with thyroid hormone. Following a piece I wrote on what appeared to be a link between synthetic thyroid hormone (Thyroxine) and increased cancer risk, I was sent a lot of information especially from America. This stated that if someone has low thyroid hormone levels they should first be immediately tested for their iodine levels as this mineral is very important in the hormone's production.

Secondly, the use of synthetic thyroid hormone is body mass dependent. So a short thin lady should not be given the same dose as a tall fat one. In America I am assured they do not, and I was told by one American doctor that they even correct for weather conditions! Three women I was talking to in the UK, all with low thyroid hormone levels, were different in size and shape. None had been tested for iodine levels. All had been given exactly the same daily thyroxine dose. All developed breast cancer. Two American doctors explained that if someone was deficient in iodine, they needed first to correct that and might not even need thyroxine supplementation. Thereafter, changes in temperature, eating shell fish or other iodine-rich foods, and over prescription of the drug Thyroxine could all result in an excess of synthetic thyroid presence and stimulate the cancer pathway.

Melatonin is a hormone produced about one and a half hours into sleep. It helps put you into a deeper sleep. It does not cause cancer; exactly the opposite. It is protective.

Many doctors think of it as a sleep aid but it is much more than that. It is the most significant antioxidant produced by the body. It is also a regulator for both oestrogen and IGF-1. Unfortunately it declines with age.

There have now been many studies covered in Cancer Watch showing that both men and women with disturbed sleep patterns develop more hormonally driven cancers. For example, studies in the USA (Harvard Medical School and Brigham) amongst both female and male night shift workers, and studies by SAS, the Scandinavian airline, on long-haul staff show that sleep deprivation causes a fall in melatonin levels and is associated with a higher risk of breast cancer in females and prostate cancer in males. Harvard Medical School also produced an analysis of the Boston Nurses Study showing that nurses on at least three night shifts a month for 15 years had a 35 per cent higher colon cancer risk.

Professor David Spiegel of Stanford University Medical Center in California, confirms that melatonin slows production of oestrogen, adding that 'sleep protects against cancer, since oestrogen is known to proliferate cancer cells'. You should always sleep in a fully darkened room with no external or synthetic light sources. Use eye shades if needs be.

But sleep deprivation is not the only cause of melatonin depletion. It can also be disturbed and depleted by Electromagnetic Frequencies or EMFs. IARC, the International Research Agency on Cancer in Lyon, France, has talked of declaring a lack of sleep as a carcinogen. But they have also presented research studies that show EMFs (from masts and aerials, mobile phones and WiFi) may deplete the hormone melatonin too. One study from Harvard Medical School even showed that EMFs could reduce the action of Tamoxifen in treating breast cancer.

We also covered the story of a block of apartments in Canada. There were 12 apartments per floor. The roof was covered with about 30 dishes and aerials. Over a three year period all bar one of the top floor apartments contained someone who had developed cancer since moving to the block.

I know of three top doctors/oncologists who take daily supplements of melatonin just before bedtime.

They know its powers. Although readily available over the counter in supermarkets in the USA, melatonin is only available on prescription in the UK and Europe and then most doctors think it is just a sleeping aid. It is best taken shortly before bedtime, 3–6 mgs being the 'normal' level taken. Over 10 mgs, it has been known to induce hallucination and startling dreams.

Only recently melatonin has been found present in red grape skins which may explain the soporific effects of red wine! Another plant melatonin is called Asphalia and is grown under Government grant.

Progesterone is a second female sex hormone. In the natural state it is a 'balancer' to oestrogen. For example, in the first half of her menstrual cycle, a woman's oestrogen levels build to the point of ovulation. Thereafter, progesterone is the lead hormone, keeping oestrogen levels in check during the second half of the cycle. Natural progesterone has the effect of balancing oestrogens in both females and males; an enzyme 'feed¬back' system determines that when too much oestrogen is produced, the production system cuts off. However, research shows that this feedback system is not affected by chemical oestrogens from external sources.

The **importance** of considering natural progesterone as a balancer to oestrogen cannot be stressed enough. They are balancing twins in the natural state. There is a significant finding from two research studies that pre-menopausal women who have breast cancer operations in the second part of their cycle (when progesterone is dominant) have a 10-¬year survival rate of 75 per cent, whereas pre¬menopausal women who have the same operation in the first two weeks of their cycle (when oestrogen is dominant) have 45 per cent 10-year survival rates. *(Imperial Cancer Research Fund, 15 Nov 1999)* The good news is that overall breast cancer survival rates have improved since the mid-nineties.

But the point is still valid. With more and more breast cancers being developed by younger women, operations should be undertaken in the second two weeks of the menstrual cycle.

It is important to understand that there is a great difference between natural and synthetic progesterone. Synthetic progesterone (more correctly called progestin in the USA and progestagen in the UK) seemingly has little or no effect on the oestrogen balancing feedback system. Worse, synthetic progesterone has a number of negative side-effects and it is linked to an increased risk of certain cancers.

In the American Women's Health Initiative study, women taking synthetic oestrogen HRT supplements had a 26 per cent increase in breast cancer. However, a combined synthetic oestrogen and progestin supplement saw a 100 per cent increased risk of breast cancer. These results caused the research study to be stopped after just three of the five years planned.

The negative publicity behind the study's findings caused a mass exodus from HRT supplementation in America and a 7 per cent decline in breast cancer cases, the first ever significant fall.

The 26 per cent figure is exactly in line with the findings of The Boston Nurses Study in the mid-nineties. Risk increases are not just confined to breast cancer. After HRT supplementation, there was an increase in colon cancer too.

A study at Johns Hopkins in Baltimore and reported in *The American Journal of Epidemiology* showed conclusively that women with lowered natural progesterone have a five and a half-fold increased risk of breast cancer and a ten-fold increased risk of any cancer.

Sherrill Sellman, an expert in female hormones, holds the view that *"Natural progesterone should oust oestrogen from centre stage."* With some justification, it would seem.

It would be fair to say that while natural progesterone is helpful in limiting oestrogen and therefore protective, synthetic progesterone has rather a lot of question marks hanging over it.

CHAPTER 3

WHAT EXACTLY IS OESTROGEN?

Oestrogen is the primary female sex hormone; a naturally occurring human steroid hormone. In fact, it is not a single hormone, but a collective name for a number of members of the same family. All are secreted typically by the ovary and, during pregnancy, by the placenta. However that is not the only source in the body. Oestrogen may be produced by the adrenal glands, the liver and the breasts. Importantly, it can also be produced in your fat stores, whether you are female or male!

As you will see, Oestrogen has the ability to create havoc in the cell; to 'mutate' the whole cell. Receptor sites on the surface are followed by a transport system that takes oestrogen molecules to the DNA In the nucleus. It also has the ability to cause cancer by triggering the production of an enzyme called AID. In small amounts this enzyme helps the immune system. However, researchers at the Cancer Research facility at Clare Hall in Hertfordshire found that at higher levels AID can cause direct DNA mutations *(Journal of Experimental Medicine; Jan 2009)*. Oestrogen has the ability to cause and spread metastases. The growth of metastases is highly dependent upon oestrogen, and the metastases in secondary regions lie dormant until oestrogen activates them *(Clin Exp Metastases, June 29, 2012, Ganapathy V et al)*.

It is also important to understand that oestrogen does not just drive cancer. Oestrogen can lie behind a host of illnesses from Polycystic Ovaries (PCOS), increasingly common in young women, to benign prostate enlargement, (BPH or BEP), increasingly common in forty-something men.

One important factor to understand is the hierarchy of danger in oestrogens:

Oestradiol is by far the most dangerous human oestrogen. It possesses the ability to sit on receptor sites located on the cell's surface and then play havoc with the cell's internal systems via its effect on the DNA in the nucleus. Its effects include affecting membrane mineral pumps so that the cell has a diminished level of potassium but an increased level of sodium. This affects the performance of the power stations (mitochondria) which then produce waste products that are more acid than normal, lowering their ability to use oxygen in an ever diminishing downward cycle. The mitochondria thus produce less and less energy as they become more and more poisoned. The *p53* gene is responsible for maintaining a normal rate of cellular growth. However, oestradiol turns off this gene by turning on the *BCL2* gene. This allows dominance in the cell of the *ras* gene which is now uncontrolled and can cause it to grow rapidly. Oestradiol then plays an important part in changing the signalling process in the cell, encouraging it to send out metastases. *(Sudipa Saha Roy, University of Texas;*

International Journal of Breast Cancer Volume 2012).

The aim with Tamoxifen, for example, is to have it sit on these same receptor sites and thus block the oestradiol from sitting there too and then doing its worst.

Oestrone, another human oestrogen, is about 40 times less powerful than oestradiol and causes considerably smaller effects inside the cell. It sits on the same receptor sites. Thus you would rather have oestrone present than oestradiol.

Certain enzymes in the body can turn dangerous oestradiol into weaker and safer oestrone and vice versa. Recent research has shown how some foods contain bioactive ingredients that can stimulate these enzymes to produce more of the safer sister oestrone. Indole 3 carbinol and its metabolite DIM do exactly that – they are found in broccoli, cabbage and Brussels sprouts, but beware over-cooking.

Phytoestrogens are plant based oestrogens and far, far weaker than human oestrogen. They have little or no negative effects on the inside of a cell. However they are less likely to sit on such receptor sites by a factor of between one hundredth and one thousandth and they are rapidly metabolised and expelled by the body. Typically, phytoestrogens come from fruits and plants, including herbs and pulses, like lentils and beans and peas, and chickpeas and kidney beans. There are three major classifications: *isoflavones* (pulses and legumes), *lignans* (whole grains and seeds) and *coumestans* (alfalfa and clover) and most of the food sources will include more than one of these three types. Lignans, for example, have anti-oestrogenic benefits at the cellular level and seem to be able to bind to fats and oestrogenic products in the blood stream and in the gut, aiding their removal from the body. Citrus isoflavones have also had some limited success with the treatment of brain tumours.

Women in South East Asia can have plasma phytoestrogen levels hundreds of times higher than their New York equivalents. Although there is some conflict in research studies, by and large higher phytoestrogen consumption seems linked with less bone fractures, less prostate growth and less breast cancer. This is hardly a surprise. For example, oestrogen is known to cause benign prostate enlargement and anti-oestrogen drugs like Finasteride and ICI have been used to reduce the size of the prostate. Phytoestrogens seem to be able to regulate the levels of human oestrogens in the body and thus limit their action in the breast, prostate and elsewhere.

Soya is a controversial subject. In 2002 Cancer Research UK published two studies, one from Singapore, the other from the NCI, concluding that women who consumed the most soya had less, risky, dense breast tissue. In 2012 research from Vanerbilt University concluded that soya consumption could prolong survival in breast cancer patients. Epidemiologists at Loma Linda University in California showed that men who drink one glass of soya milk a day have a 30 per cent lower risk of prostate cancer; more than one glass sees this figure rise to 70 per cent.

However, soya is an incomplete protein containing no vitamin B-12, for example, and the rapid increase of soya milk consumption in the West has been associated with allergies and dietary problems.

Soya milk is a red herring. People wishing to beat cancer should avoid cows' milk consumption as it increases inflammation and IGF-1 levels. But I'm not 100 per cent sure they should switch to consuming vast amounts of soya milk either. Personally I am extremely concerned about the high levels of GMO soya, especially in American products and I would not touch it, for that reason alone.

However, soya beans are pulses along with other beans and peas and lentils. They are but one example of phytoestrogens. Soy contains isoflavones such as genistein, and fermented soya products have been long associated with health.

The National Cancer Institute has confirmed that there are anti-tumour properties in the herb red clover, which has ten times the genistein content of soy. Georgetown University Medical School in Washington has confirmed that genistein helps repair proteins with damaged DNA; and according to the NCI, genistein helps prevent tumours from developing blood supplies.

Just ask yourself, 'Which would I rather have? Oestradiol sitting on my cellular receptor sites, or phytoestrogens from plants, fruits and pulses?

At the Royal Marsden Professor Trevor Powles attempted to find out whether genistein could have the same action as Tamoxifen and prevent cancer by blocking oestrogen receptor sites. Unfortunately, he was unsuccessful in determining the exact quantity required.

Xenoestrogens are external chemicals that, once inside the body, can mimic the action of human oestrogens. A by-product of this modern world, they are a class of environmental pollutants which may be ingested or breathed, and can be found in pesticides, herbicides, exhaust, solvents like nail polish remover and nail polish, liquid soaps, cosmetics, toys, white liners in cans and plastic water bottles. They can also be found in water supplies, along with the remains of the contraceptive pill, HRT and certain drugs which are hormone disruptive. They cause many general sexual problems.

For example, research from Mount Sinai School of Medicine in New York with over a thousand young girls showed that phenols (for example, Bisphenol A, or BPA) and phthalates both hastened puberty. Mary Wolff, the lead researcher said that the research showed a link between the chemicals girls were exposed to on a daily basis, and early development.

Phthalates are a class of chemicals used widely in plastic and vinyl to make packaging, especially plastic packaging, furniture, inks, soft plastics for toys, cosmetics adhesives, detergents and even sex toys!

The University of Rochester showed such chemicals could alter levels of male hormone formation in boys still in the womb; phthalates were found to alter the production of testosterone.

Between 2002 and 2007, several studies took place in America on a common herbicide called Atrazine after it was noted that populations of male frogs in the fields were developing female characteristics. Researcher Dr Tyrone B Hayes of UCLA Berkeley said that it was dangerous at very low levels. *"If you take 5 grains of salt, and divide this weight by 5,000, that is still strong enough to give male frogs ovaries"*, he said. The herbicide is widely used throughout the world to 'treat' crops such as sugar cane, macadamia nuts, maize and pineapples. *"There is no Atrazine-free area in the environment"*, he added.

Oestrogen is also used in farming to encourage animals to gain weight, and it is now known that xenoestrogens can disrupt glucose metabolism, increase the risk of diabetes and encourage weight gain in humans.

Xenoestrogens are chemicals you should do your best to avoid!

CHAPTER 4

WHAT ELSE IS IMPORTANT TO KNOW ABOUT OESTROGEN?

Every day, each of us produces 200 or more pre-cancer cells as a result of our normal lives. Usually, our immune systems are more than capable of neutralising all of these. However, members of the oestrogen family act as a cancer helper, fanning the flames of cancer in the body and helping cancer overwhelm the defensive systems.

It is not the intention of this book to duplicate others I have written, nor to give long, detailed explanations of the cancer process. Suffice it here to make a couple of relevant points.

Experts in cancer all over the world are not 100 per cent certain or agreed on exactly how cancers start. Typically a simple statement of DNA damage or mutation is trotted out. Yes, radiation damage from nuclear fallout can cause cancer. But after that? Your cancer is as individual as you are - I've been saying this for ten years. Now Cancer Research has proved it. Research on 1400 cases of breast cancer found that no two cancers were the same. Another CRUK study showed that you could group breast cancer alone into at least ten sub-groups.

In cancer, genes go wrong and fail to produce certain key chemicals like proteins. In prostate cancer 5,900 genes were shown to be working abnormally. Thirteen external chemicals have been shown to be gene-disruptive in this picture.

Cancer cells are different – they are rapidly dividing, out of control, anaerobic (they do not derive their energy using oxygen) and the centre of tumours is extremely acidic (about 6.2 pH). They also try to take over your normal, healthy body systems. So for example, the energy production system (now confined to the area outside of the non-functioning power stations) burns glucose in the absence of oxygen. The waste product is lactic acid, similar to that involved in cramp in sportsmen. The lactic acid is dealt with in the liver before it causes tissue damage. The waste product of this is glucose, which passes back round the body to feed the cancer. Cancer may attack your bones. The bones produce growth hormone to strengthen themselves. The cancer uses this to grow a blood supply and grow into a bigger tumour. The cancer produces chemicals that affect your adrenal glands causing them to produce more cortisol. This in turn causes more inflammation and increases acidity in tissues all over the body. It makes metastases easier. And so on.

The bottom line if you want to beat cancer? Don't worry about the detail – take charge of the things you can control:

* The causes that may still be driving your cancer – and oestrogen is very likely to be one of those;

* The various steps in the cancer process known to be affected by bioactive compounds; *'The Rainbow Diet'* addresses these (for example, talking about the

benefits of phenols like curcumin, or resveratrol, or vitamin D and fish oils which should be included in all anti-cancer programmes),

* And rebuilding a healthy new 'you'. *'Everything you need to know to help you beat cancer'* includes a useful programme, (for example, restoring a healthy gut, avoiding glucose and cows' dairy, taking light daily exercise etc)

So let's get back to dealing with oestrogen.

Oestrogen can be made in your fat stores

Oestrogen is known to be made from fat stores in the body. Firstly, it is known that female athletes with low levels of body fat often have a loss of menstrual cycles. Conversely women with a high percentage of body fat (over 25 - 28 per cent) also have direct reproductive consequences

(a) Adipose tissue converts androgens to oestrogen by the action of an enzyme called aromatase, making body fat a significant source of oestrogen.

(b) body weight, hence fatness, influences the direction of oestrogen metabolism to more potent or less potent forms; leaner women make more catechol oestrogens like oestrone, the less potent form;

(c) obese women and young, fat girls have a diminished capacity for oestrogen to bind sex-hormone binding-globulin and so 'free' oestrogen is higher in the blood stream;

(d) adipose tissue can store steroid hormones. *(Source:*

MMR, *Oxford Journals)*

Fat is an excellent solvent and your fat stores will hold hormones, for example your own and/or synthetic ones from pesticides and chemicals of concern in personal care products, that you would rather have excreted.

As already mentioned, this fits with the 2012 American Cancer Society report that weight control will increase survival and even prevent a cancer returning. The good news is that there is research from Northwestern Medical School showing that it is never too late to start your weight control programme. Women with breast cancer increased their survival times the more they reduced their weight to appropriate levels.

What else should I know about oestrogen?

Oestrogen is known to lower levels of folic acid in the body. Folic acid is a B vitamin essential to the correct copying process of your DNA and RNA. With low levels, mistakes can occur; mistakes that could lead to cancer forming.

Oestrogen and oestrogen mimics encourage the body to put on weight, and fat.

Oestrogen can help cancer grow and spread. As Professor David Spiegel stated earlier, we know oestrogen proliferates cancer cells. It causes more and more to be made.

So oestrogen is implicated in both cancer cause, and cancer spread. And it is not just breast cancer risk that increases with oestrogen levels. For example:

1. According to US research *(May 2005, Cancer Research)*, **lung cancer** cells grow in response to oestrogen, and researchers showed that a drug, gefitnib, could block the pathway by which oestrogen worked.

2. Women on the contraceptive pill have twice the risk of **melanoma** (Harvard Medical School, 1999) than their identical peers not on the pill. *Feskanich et al* have stated that 'oestrogens can increase melanocyte and melatonin count and cause hyper-pigmentation of the skin.'

3. Some **brain tumours** have been linked to oestrogen toxins *(NCI)*.

4. Oestrogen actually contributes to **colon cancer,** and localised oestrogen production may again be the key. So says M. English and team at the University of Birmingham and reported in August 2000 in *The British Journal of Cancer.*

5. Dr Carol Rosenberg of Evanston-Northwestern Healthcare, USA published a study of 92,835 post¬menopausal women in December 2003. In the study, 25 per cent of those who developed mild skin cancer went on to get a second different cancer later, against a 'norm' of 11 per cent. Interestingly the skin cancers and the second cancers could all be counted as 'oestrogen driven'.

Cancer Research UK has shown that levels of oestrogen are increasing, on average, in females by about seven per cent a year.

OESTROGEN. *The Killer in our Midst*

CHAPTER 5
BREAKTHROUGH, REVOLUTIONARY THINKING

In November 2004, Professor Timothy Wang and his team at Columbia University reported their 'breakthrough' research in *Science*.

Wang and his team were looking at stomach cancer. Firstly, they noted that problems always started with inflammation in the stomach wall. Next, they noted that stem cells from the bone marrow rushed to the site of the inflammation to heal it.

What are stem cells? A very, very simplistic explanation might be to imagine a fertilised egg growing in the mother's womb. For the first 50 or so days, this is a 'blob' of rapidly multiplying cells. Not until day 54-56 does this blob of cells slow down its division and 'differentiate' into finger, toe, eye, liver, heart and other specialist cells.

For 'blob' of cells, read stem cells!

You have stem cells throughout your body and throughout your life. They are your repair cells, waiting to transform themselves into whatever cell is required. Without them we would not heal, nor would we make new eye cells, or liver cells. Every day we have a high turnover of cells in each of us.

Stem cells are rather like cancer cells in that they multiply rapidly, and also they do not die.

They invade an inflamed or damaged area and convert into cells of the type required. In scientific terms it is called differentiation. Thus ordinarily, Wang would have expected the repair stem cells to become new stomach wall cells.

However in his research, he observed that the stem cells rushed to the inflammation but that, **under the influence of localised oestrogen,** they did not convert into new stomach cells but stayed as rapidly multiplying, non-dying cells. And thus a cancer had started. The report stated that this new research would mean that *'the orthodox textbooks on the causes of cancer would need to be re-written'*.

Well done to Professor Wang. But there's one slight problem: his revolutionary theory was a mere 98 years old!

Back in 1906 a Mancunian embryologist, John Beard, working in Edinburgh noted that the 'blob' of undifferentiated cells in the foetus divided rapidly under the influence of oestrogen. He further noticed that, around day 54-56 when the cells switched over to normal cells, the foetus suddenly had pancreatic, or digestive, enzymes present. Since its food already came 'pre-prepared' from its mother, he hypothesised that these enzymes were, in fact, doing a different job. They were converting the blob of rapidly dividing stem cells into eye, liver, kidney, brain, heart cells and more.

He wrote papers back in 1906 about his theory of cancer: Put simply, stem cells are held back by oestrogen in a 'trophoblastic' state and become cancer cells. Pancreatic (or digestive) enzymes could switch off this process making them 'normal'. He then went a little further. Since stem cells exist all over the body, for example in the breast tissue or the prostate tissue, he said that a cancer was rather like having a baby growing in the wrong place at the wrong time! Not surprisingly, he was laughed at and his work forgotten about.

I was outlining this slightly bizarre story at a speech in the UK and hypothesising that, if true, we would not need any expensive new tests for predicting each cancer. A highly sensitive pregnancy test would show the answer; even for men.

A woman in the audience stood up and said, *"I have to interrupt you. I'm 39 and last year I felt so ill I thought I must be pregnant. So I did two self-tests and I was. I went to the Doctor and he confirmed it. However, three months later, instead, he identified I wasn't pregnant; I had breast cancer!"*

One positive end product of the Beard work is that, in the New York clinic of Dr. Nicholas Gonzalez, cancer patients are being treated with some success using large numbers of supplements including pancreatic enzymes. He even ran his own clinical trial.

Cancer Stem Cells

Since Wang there has been an eight year argument between opposite groups of scientists, one arguing that cancer stem cells lay at the heart of all cancer tumours; the other group arguing it was rubbish. In 2012 there were three major studies showing the cancer stem cell theory was true, and scientists at Cancer Research UK even isolated them.

For example, Professor Hugo Snippert of Utrecht Medical School said that normal tissues had healthy cells at their centre, while cancers had cancer stem cells at their centre. A cause for concern was the quote from one research group (Luis Parada and his team from University of Texas Southwestern Medical School) who add that there was no current drug available that could kill cancer stem cells. Existing drugs could reduce a tumour by 30, 50 even 70 per cent, a fact Parada described as 'irrelevant'. The risk was always there that the tumour could re-grow. In 2012 and 13 there were numerous studies concluding the cancer stem cell theory was correct in cancers from prostate to multiple myeloma. Parada added, *'At least now we know exactly what job we need to tackle'.*

But hope is at hand. Also in 2012 Dr Young S Kim, working for the National Cancer Institute in Bethesda, showed that 'bad foods' could cause the cancer to re-grow, but bioactive ingredients found in a variety of natural compounds could prevent that re-growth. She named sulphoraphanes (typically in sprouting seeds and broccoli) curcumin, piperine (black pepper), vitamin A and complete vitamin E, theanine and choline, genistein (red clover), and EGCG (green tea) as very important adding that you could find all of these in supplements *(Kim et al., Journal of Nutritional Biochemistry; July 2012).*

So, in conclusion, here we have a theory on how oestrogen may be responsible for many more cancers.

CHAPTER 6
WHAT HAS OESTROGEN GOT TO DO WITH MEN AND THEIR CANCERS?

Men get prostate cancer and testicular cancer. And they have melanoma, colon cancer and brain tumours too. Virtually all prostate cancers are thought to be hormonally responsive and caused largely by age-related changes in the androgen/oestrogen balance. Androgens are the male sex hormones. Many men with prostate cancer will have been advised that they have too much testosterone and this is the cause of their cancer. **This can be extremely misleading.** There is absolutely no scientific evidence that testosterone causes cancer of any sort. Nor is there any scientific evidence that testosterone **spreads** cancer. It may well be that many men who have prostate cancer also have high testosterone levels, just as they may have more dentures or thinning hair, but it is not the primary CAUSE or the factor that SPREADS it.

Logically, if high testosterone levels alone were the cause of prostate cancer every red-blooded eighteen year old male would have it. Testosterone as the cause of prostate cancer? Pure myth and nonsense.

The National Cancer Centre in Singapore have looked at factors that can stop the spread of prostate cancer, and they have shown that anti-oestrogens (e.g. ICI and Finasteride) both reduced spread and growth (by up to 50 per cent) of the prostate cells.

Research findings are clear that oestrogen (human and/or chemical) in men is associated with a variety of issues, from increasing prostate size, to increasing prostate cancer risk, to increasing testicular cancer risk, to suppressing sperm levels *(Handlesman et al; Concord Hospital, Sydney; March 2002)*. Several studies have directly linked oestrogen mimics to declining sperm count. Oestrogen mimics like BPA have been shown to lower testosterone levels directly.

Research from the Monash Institute, Victoria, Australia *(Risbridger, Bianco et al)* concluded that **prostate cancer is caused by localised production of oestrogens.** The research concludes that only androgen (e.g. testosterone) **when combined with oestrogen** produces malignancy and that neither hormone alone is sufficient to produce it. Doctor Ian Thompson of the MD Anderson Cancer Center in Texas stated that *"Finasteride (an anti-oestrogen) is the first drug that has been shown to reduce the risk of prostate cancer"*. Thompson went further. He believes oestrogens stimulate the conversion of 'harmless' testosterone into the real active problem, dihydrotestosterone (DHT), a very potent hormone.

Although this conversion normally occurs due to human oestrogen, indeed oestradiol, it has been shown that chemicals that mimic the action of oestrogen, once in the body, can most certainly play a part.

Natural progesterone has been shown to have some effect as a 'limiter' of prostate growth and prostate cancer. Whilst synthetic progestagen may be given to prostate sufferers to curb their 'testosterone' levels, it will simultaneously inhibit their oestrogen levels too. So, this could well be a case of 'right drug – wrong reason!'

Of course, some prostate cancer sufferers are actually treated by using oestrogen supplementation. This 'works' for a while because if you throw huge volumes of oestrogen into the male body, testosterone levels fall to near zero, so no DHT can be made. This therapy will work providing the theory of homeostasis does not hold true – i.e. eventually the body will try to rebalance and produce at least some testosterone. Unfortunately, the testosterone fights back.

Oestrogen supplementation as a prostate cancer therapy may increase blood clotting risk.

One 2012/3 research study followed the observations that broccoli (and thus indole 3 carbinol and DIM, plus sulphoraphanes) could at least slow down the progression of prostate cancer (by denaturing oestradiol and affecting the binding sites), while other research showed more phenol bioactive compounds in pomegranate, curcumin and green tea (EGCG) could be of benefit. Professor Robert Thomas in the UK conducted clinical trials on a supplement containing all of these, which he called Pomi-T, showing that it reduced PSA levels by 60 per cent.

Men make oestrogen in a variety of ways as they age, not least of all by being overweight. Fat makes steroids, makes oestrogen. Low levels of exercise do not help. One US study concluded that some overweight 55-year old men could have higher oestrogen levels than their

35-year old girlfriends! Of course there are other ways men increase their oestrogen pools. They have started to use large volumes of perfumed toiletries; they consume pesticides, are surrounded by chemicals and household cleaners; they may consume too much red, hormone-fed, meat and/or sleep badly and/or be too close to powerful EMFs. They may also drink too much alcohol. Alcohol certainly does not help beat prostate cancer. It is a carcinogen which increases blood glucose levels and fat stores. Put that pint of beer down! Interestingly, research from the Wake Forest Cancer Institute, Carolina (published BJC, 13 October 2003) concludes that a gene CYP1B1 is linked to your susceptibility to prostate cancer. The gene has 13 variants, of which certain variants were found to respond to environmental toxins that were xenoestrogens.

Resveratrol, a natural compound found in grape skins, can affect this CYP1B1 gene and Professors Potter and Burke have studied a number of bioactive foods which they say have the same effect. The CYP1B1 gene acts on the resveratrol and turns it into a compound which selectively kills the cancer cell. Potter and Burke have developd these Bioactive foods into compounds they call Salvestrols - and they have research showing Salvestrols can stop hormone-driven cancers.

The reason oestrogen is 'linked' to breast cancer so publicly and less to prostate, colon or melanoma is simply the volume of funding raised and therefore research being done on breast cancer compared with the others and then the extra PR it all gets in the papers.

But the fact is that oestrogen plays its part in male cancers too. And the action is very similar to that occurring in women's cancers.

CHAPTER 7
CHEMICAL MIMICS
OF OESTROGEN

I continually mention xenoestrogens. These are hormone disruptive chemicals found in pesticides, herbicides, plastics, vinyls, cosmetics, personal care products and toiletry products, children's plastic toys, flame-proofed chairs, household cleaners and much more. Once in the blood stream, they can mimic the action of the oestrogen family.

So, they can be called oestrogen mimics, endocrine disrupters, hormone disrupters, gender benders or xenoestrogens.

Cancer – the modern disease

In the 1940's the world produced 1 million tonnes of chemicals. Now that figure is over 600 million tonnes.

Cancer is a modern disease. *The National Geographic News* (July 13th, 2004) confirms this. A study of over 3000 human skeletons dating back to 5300 BC by US scientists in Croatia hardly turned up one case of cancer before the middle of the 19th century.

As Professor Trevor Powles of the Royal Marsden, Surrey, England, said in his 2004 interview with **icon**, *"principally, I think breast cancer has increased because of environmental reasons (including oestrogens and other agents/ chemicals in the food), and intake of hormones like HRT and oral*

41

contraceptives." And he should know. At the time he was the top man in the UK on breast cancer!

Common plastic packaging

An infamous anecdote concerns Dr Ana Soto of Tufts Cancer Centre in the USA who was growing cancer cells in what were normally glass jars by stimulating them with oestrogen. When she blocked the oestrogen the cancer cells stopped growing. But suddenly after a considerable dormant period, even without added oestrogen, she noticed that they were growing again. Then she found that the glass jars had been replaced by plastic ones and the plastic was leaching oestrogen-like chemicals into her test cells.

The World Health Organisation wants governments to ban two common elements of plastic packaging - phthalates and BPA. They are plasticisers used to harden plastic. Women with a history of miscarriages have higher levels of bisphenol A in their bloodstreams *(Nagoya Medical School, Japan)*.

You can find them in plastic water bottles containing healthy spring water, plastic wraps over sandwiches, white linings inside cans and more. And do not be fooled into thinking that thick plastic bottles are safer than thin as some people opine. It all depends on the types of plasticisers used. Some plasticisers leach hormone disrupters, some don't.

Plastic thermos beakers were shown to leach more hormone-disrupters once they had had hot liquids in them; the heat denatured the plastic. Even in subsequent cold drinks, the hormone-disrupter chemicals were higher than before the hot drinks had been present. Even plastic water bottles left in the sunshine in a car suffer the fate of increasing the leached levels. And so does your suntan cream on the beach.

Mind you, it also may well contain chemicals such as oxybenzone, retinyl palmitate and a well established xenoestrogen, 4-methylbenzylidene, which can increase localised oestrogen levels on the skin. The Environmental Working Group in America claims only one in five sunscreens is truly safe, as localised oestrogen is a driver of skin cancer and melanoma.

Safe limits?

'But there are safe limits set by our governments', I hear you cry! Three points are relevant here:

Firstly, the governments of the world are inconsistent. Formaldehyde is banned in Sweden and Japan, but in the UK, Australia and the USA your shampoos, nail polishes and household cleaners are likely to contain it in one form or another (it comes under about forty different names). Canada has banned BPA completely; France wants to do the same in 2015. California has banned it from toys for children under three years of age. But plastic baby feeding bottles can be culprits throughout Europe.

Most governments have quite simply ignored the report from the World Health Organisation asking them to urgently ban hormone-disrupters like BPA, phthalates and parabens mentioned above.

Euro MPs passed a resolution to ban over 1,000

chemicals of concern in everyday products. A ban was reconsidered. Instead, a project which will take at least 15 years to complete is looking at these chemicals one by one and also examining safer alternatives. Johnson and Johnson has decided to lead the way in the high streets by removing six or more chemicals of concern from baby products and others.

Secondly, what is a safe level? As I said at the start of the book, hormones can work at levels of one part in a trillion. Yet some 'safe' limits for ingredients are set as one part in a million by government health authorities. So these chemical ingredients will be in your bloodstream at thousands of times larger levels than even your most powerful hormones!

Finally, what if all these different xenoestrogens merely accumulated in your body, so there were, quite simply, no safe limits? Dr. Ana Soto of Tufts took just ten such ingredients, all at government approved safe limits, and showed a full oestrogen response in her test animals. These xenoestrogens are cumulative.

Cheryl Watson and her team at the University of Texas Medical Branch in Galvaston showed in 2013 that three oestrogen mimics (BPA, the supposedly safer BPS and a nonylphenol which is commonly used in household detergents), had both a cumulative and interactive effect. They affect pituitary cells at parts per quadrillion! This is very disturbing because your pituitary is the boss of your endocrine system and even controls chemical reactions such as cell division in your body.

The growing chemical time bomb

A UK Royal Commission has concluded that you are likely to come across about 4,000 chemical ingredients in the average month, many of which are toxic. USA research shows that women who use considerably more products (face creams, lipsticks, eye shadows, hair dyes, cleansers etc, etc.) than their men, have four times the level of such toxins in their bloodstreams.

In Australia, I met a number of farmers who blamed their own leukaemia and multiple myeloma on the pesticides they themselves used. A link between multiple myeloma and pesticides has been established. Farmers do have higher rates of the disease and it is linked to the pesticides causing 'sticky' proteins, termed MUGS, in the blood.

Then there are water supplies. IARC has talked about herbicides and pesticides running off the fields into water supplies. Nitrates and nitrites, not just gender bending chemicals, are linked to brain and kidney cancer. Water purification systems in cities cannot cope with the rapid advancement in drugs. Research has shown recycled city water contains drugs, antibiotics, sweeteners like aspartame, and oestrogen from HRT and contraceptive pills.

The Contamination study by WWF found an average of 27 chemicals in the blood of the UK citizens tested, including PCBs and DDT, out of a list of 77 highly toxic chemicals they looked for.

A second report on 80 ingredients concluded matters were worsening. Our parents had 56 ingredients, on average, in their bloodstreams.

Meanwhile our children have, on average, 75 of the 80 in theirs.

US Centers for Disease Control and Prevention started analysing the blood of thousands of Americans in 1999. Over the years they have shown that this *'toxic burden'* is growing and enormous. Our bodies and organs like the liver simply do not 'recognise' these new chemicals which have developed since the Second World War, and so these chemicals are not metabolised but simply pushed around the body until they are stored in your fat deposits.

Next, there is the *'chemical reaction'* problem. Twenty chemicals stored together might react causing the production of other chemicals. Far-fetched? Researchers at the University of Liverpool in 2005 showed that aspartame, MSG and two food colouring agents could react in the body and kill nerve cells. So that could be some junk snacks and a can of diet drink! It's a health time bomb.

Be clear. We are not talking only about cancer here. Chemical toxins in the body have been linked to a raft of degenerative, chronic diseases. The two groups of chemicals called dioxins and acrylamides have, according to health authorities like the WHO and the FDA, no safe levels.

Hormone disrupted mutants?

There are also hormone disrupters you breathe. **Volatile organic carbons** (VOCs) are harmful chemicals given off readily by a number of everyday substances. For example, petrol fumes when filling your car; glues used to attach floor or ceiling tiles or to stick together cheaper wood products; inks used by faxes, gases from the circuitry of computers; gases from bleaches and all manner of household cleaners and disinfectants, dry cleaning and chlorine products. Most paper products are treated with chlorine and can give off gases or be absorbed through your hands. Toxins linked to cancer abound in our everyday lives.

Carpets hold and encourage air dust and so the gases join with the dust particles and are inhaled. Hungarian and Austrian scientists (**icon** September 2003) showed that these toxins collect at the crossroads in the air passages at 400 times the levels elsewhere.

In the WWF study, the most common contaminants in children were:

1. **Polychlorinated biphenyls** from coolants, flame-retardants and plastics: known to affect the nervous system and linked to liver and brain cancers.
2. **Organochlorides** from plant pesticides to mosquito repellents: linked to male genital problems and hormone disruptive, oestrogen mimic effects.
3. **Perfluorinated** chemicals from fast food packaging, non-stick utensils, stain resistant carpets and furniture polishes - linked to bladder cancer.
4. **Phthalates** from plastics in bottles to childrens' toys, and many toiletry bottles - known oestrogen

mimics and hormone disrupters.

5. **Polybrominated Diphenyl Ethers** found in flame-retardants in cars, furniture and TVs, and in clothing treatments: cause severe hormone disruption and blood disorders.

Many of these are hormone-disruptive.

Researchers have shown fish off the coast of California became hermaphrodite from the effluent reaching the sea; a second study showed much the same problem in the Potomac River just outside Washington DC. Like the frogs mentioned earlier, the gender bending chemicals are quite simply creating mutants.

Multiple studies with xenoestrogens and rodents have shown that exposure to xenoestrogens in the womb is associated to increased levels of testicular cancer in young adults and elevated levels of prostate cancer later in life. Dr David Zava of ZRT Laboratory in Oregon has a database tracking blood test results of males with prostate cancer and consistently finds lower testosterone levels but higher oestrogen and xenoestrogen levels.

Dr Philippa Darbre (Reading University) has linked breast cancer in men and women to antiperspirants *(Journal of Applied Toxicology)*. There is toluene, a xenoestrogen, in many nail polishes and perfumes. Your brain can accumulate toxins as it is very fatty. Girls in nail salons in the USA have eight times the levels of brain tumours found in normal adults.

Perfumes can contain 150 different chemicals that

do not have to be named as secrecy is part of their mystique – so too are xenoestrogens! Swedish research results in 2003 showed that two thirds of a list of perfumed products, ranging from perfumes themselves, to shampoos, deodorants, body sprays and hair colourings contained chemicals that, once inside the blood stream, were oestrogen mimics. One in particular, DEHP, when found in pregnant women is known to cause genital abnormalities in their unborn male offspring – including higher rates of testicular cancer. **Never put perfumed products on your skin.**

One important fact to consider is that **the bulk of the problem lies inside your own home**, from cleaners to plastic furniture and ceiling tile glues to chipboard products. If you go out to work, factories have pollution rules and guidelines about what can and cannot be used in the work place. But at home a woman is allowed to clean to her heart's content, using dichlorobenzene products (you know, the ones that make your toilet smell like a mountain pine forest) and formaldehyde (a Class A carcinogen) everywhere. Please read the updated article *'As safe as houses'* in the Appendix carefully and take action to go toxin-free tomorrow!

Build your own safer micro-environment

Now, before you despair, let's consider what we have learned. Much of this is avoidable in the first place. You can buy good quality water -filters, (I have an excellent system at home), you can clean up your house, you can grow and/or buy organic vegetables, you can buy toxin-free cosmetics and toiletries (Neways is a company that has kicked out over 3,000 chemicals of concern over the years). You can clean up your act.

Next, you can detox. By this, I do not mean rushing out and buying some herbal drink. The idea of a detox has been taken to completely new levels with specialist clinics and blood testing laboratories in America, Australia, Germany and the UK to mention just four countries with high standards. The Acu-Chem laboratory in Dallas is just such a place. Blood analysis will identify chemical contaminants and places such as the Hippocrates Health Institute in Florida provide three to four week programmes involving raw organic food diets, daily saunas and exercise, and the use of supplements such as selenium, multi-strain probiotics, chlorella and broccoli/indole 3 carbinol. Levels of chemicals in the blood fall dramatically. In one research study covered in Cancer Watch about 7 years ago, children whose blood held chemicals of concern took about five days to improve markedly, simply by going onto a raw, organic food diet.

CHAPTER 8
THE MICROBIOME -

WORKING TO REMOVE YOUR OESTROGEN

Two reports, one in *Science,* the other in *Nature*, both early in 2012, sounded a warning siren in America that maybe, just maybe, orthodox medicine was causing more than a few problems with the bacteria that live in and around your body. And maybe, just maybe, these are important to your perfect health. One report covered research on *Clostridium difficile.* Apparently 14,000 people die every year in hospitals in America due to *C. difficile* infections. In desperation, scientists tried an experiment. They gave seriously ill patients an enema made from the stools of healthy people. Many really sick people became better in less than 24 hours.

What's it all about? In your gut alone, you have some 800 strains of bacteria, 400 have been classified and named. About 25 come up regularly in research studies which number over 5,000 in the last five or so years. There are about a hundred clinical trials. When you were a young child, your parents thought your runny nose and fatigue was just another cold. It wasn't. You had stroked the cat and put your fingers in your mouth. The new bacteria went to your gut. The immune system responded to the new threat with antibody production and a temperature. American research concludes that as much as 85 per cent of your immune system is driven by this reaction system to relatively harmless invaders. And that is the basis of your long-term immune memory. As long as the new bacterium stays in your gut, there will be antibodies in your body. When something nastier comes along, your immune system has a head start.

The bacteria are important to your very existence. You help them by feeding them and providing a nice warm, dark environment. In turn they help protect you. Children brought up on farms have a better immune system for life, as do children brought up with household animals. That is, until you do something to harm them, like take antibiotics or certain drugs. Three weeks of antibiotics is used to kill every bacterium in mice when scientists are conducting experiments! What if the antibiotics you take kill off the bacterium you received from the cat? And what if it was simply a bacterium similar to but weaker than *C.difficile*? By killing the 'cat bacterium' off, you lose your immune protection for when something really nasty comes along. How could you defeat it? But when given the stool of a healthy person containing the 'cat bacterium', you just might be able to put up a fight.

Gut bacteria do so much more. At night when you sleep they consume yeasts like *candida albicans* and microbes that came on your food throughout the day. They love *candida*; and so they are your first line of defence. If yeasts and microbes take control in your gut, chronic inflammation can occur, with some of the parasites even entering your blood system.

Next, the good bacteria help cut up your food

working with your enzymes in a multitude of complex chemical reactions. It's why acidity in the stomach from too much salt, or alcohol, or too many pickled foods causes a problem. Changing the acidity or alkalinity of the gut from normal accelerates or, more likely, impairs the chemical reactions that release goodness and nourishment. Mind you, the foods you consume have to have the nourishment in them to release! Whole foods, fibrous foods, grains and greens are foods these bacteria adore - vitamin K from your greens; folic acid, biotin and B-12 from your grains, each helping the fight against cancer and other diseases.

But at the same time, the bacteria are taking waste products from your system and binding them to the fibre and lignans, so they can be excreted from the body. This process, called chelation, eliminates heavy metals and dangerous chemicals from your body - like nitrosamines (known to be linked to colon cancer) and oestrogenic chemicals, whether human or synthetic.

So, to remove the oestrogens from your body eat lots of fibrous foods and ensure your gut bacteria are in tip top condition at the right alkalinity/acidity.

And this is the **Microbiome**. Not surprisingly, it seems to get ill first; then you get ill. If it doesn't like certain poisons, you probably won't either – you have been living side by side as symbiotes for thousands of years. You like and hate the same things. And by the way, their enemies, yeasts, love sugar, whether from added glucose, cakes, refined pasta, ice cream, chocolate or that fruit smoothie you made yourself and drank after your lunch.

And in America they have concluded that you cannot get better until your bacteria get better. They have to get well first. It is a huge finding, one that has many oncologists extremely concerned.

Of course, you can attack your yeasts in the gut with old fashioned remedies like sodium bicarbonate (a teaspoon in warm water first thing in the morning might help). Holland and Barratt have a product called Dida, which contains all the herbs that weaken yeasts, like pau d'arco, garlic, oregano, cinnamon and more. You can boost your beneficial bacteria content with products like Probiota 7, Yakult (containing the unique *L. Casei shirota* bacterium), and Neways protozymes. Those three products will boost about ten strains. But will they replace the 'cat bacterium', or is that lost forever? Who knows? It's a real worry.

I have written much more about the microbiome and how it is linked to illnesses like MS, Arthritis, Alzheimer's and Diabetes in a new book called *'The Secret Source of your Good Health'*.

CHAPTER 9

THE OESTROGEN POOL

- A SUMMARY OF PROBLEMS

So, every one of us has a 'pool' of oestrogen in our bodies. This pool in the twenty-first century is made up from our own natural oestrogens, plus plant oestrogens and synthetic oestrogens that we ingest (from foods, water, the contraceptive pill, HRT etc.), plus a cocktail of other chemicals that find their way into our bodies and, once there, can 'mimic' the action of natural oestrogens. So let us recap this. The pool comes because:

1. You ingest more of it.
- Oestrogens which are the animal's natural hormones come with all meats.
- Some animals have oestrogen and growth hormones added.
- Oestrogen can be found in recycled tap water.
- You use the pill and/or HRT.

2. You make more of it yourself.
- Alcohol consumption raises oestrogen levels.
- Fat consumption increases oestrogen production.
- Large carbohydrate-rich meals stimulate insulin production, which in turn stimulates oestrogen levels.

- Our own fat stores can produce oestrogen

3. You store it.

- Fat is a wonderful solvent; if you are overweight you will store excess oestrogen that you should be excreting.
- Modern diets do not contain enough natural fibre to ensure excess oestrogen is properly excreted.
- You damage the deal you have with the bacteria that could have helped eliminate it from your body (You eat too much salt, and vinegary foods, drink too much alcohol: you feed their enemies with sugar, you kill the good guys with antibiotics and certain drugs, even in city water and the animals you eat).

4. You put yourself into a poor micro-environment.

For example:
- You eat foods covered in pesticides, e.g. DDT and Lindane.
- You surround yourself with toxic chemicals like volatile organic carbons at home (in glues, computer circuitry, bleaches, toiletries, detergents)
- You drink and eat from plastic cups, bottles, white lined cans (BPA and phthalates from plastics industry).
- You use products that contain parabens.
- You have lots of appliances: polychlorinated biphenyls (PCBs) e.g. used in electronics manufacturing.

- You use nail polish and cleaners, and put perfumed products on your skin.

Male or female, oestrogen and its synthetic mimics, are a modern and increasing hazard.

CHAPTER 10
FOR THE AVOIDANCE OF DOUBT

1. Our oestrogenic animals:

Compared to our ancestors, we eat more meat. With the animal's protein and fat comes the animal's natural hormones (including oestrogen) plus any that may have been artificially added to help it grow.

Furthermore, with the animal's fat come hormones like oestrogen, plus all the stored toxins and chemicals the animal has picked up from the pesticide and herbicide residues in the fields; plus the plethora of injections, antibiotics and growth enhancers (and even hormones) given to make it stronger, bigger and infection-resistant. Yummy! Even your nice safe chicken breast is likely to have residues of antibiotics if not organic chicken.

Over 480 herbicides, pesticides and animal growth and 'protective' chemicals are legally permitted in farming in the USA, of which some two thirds have been shown to be directly or indirectly carcinogenic. 82 chemicals are legally permitted for animals alone. Britain is not far behind. And a large number of the pesticide residues, once they have entered our bodies, can 'mimic' oestrogen.

In an earlier chapter I told the story of Israel and DDT and Lindane getting in to the food chain with calamitous results. The problem for you and I is that when Western Governments banned such infamous pesticides, they only banned their local use. The same companies still manufacture DDT but sell it abroad. Third World countries then grow their vegetables, use the pesticides and export the produce back to us!! Moreover, there are still many, many pesticides used in our countries whose effects are not fully known.

The good news is that the **New York Medical College has shown that curcumin can reduce the effects of DDT in the body, has anti-oestrogenic effects and is synergistic with phytoestrogens.**

2. Adding Oestrogen through drugs:

When the contraceptive pill was first introduced there was only one study performed which could be called a proper clinical trial and that showed clear risks in taking it. Despite this, a large dose oestrogen pill was launched for women. Fortunately, in the seventies and eighties levels of oestrogen were reduced in the pill as more links to cancer were found.

In 2002 Cancer Research UK figures showed the following increased risk of breast cancer for women taking oestrogen-based contraceptive pills.

Ever taken	+ 26 per cent
Taken into their 30s	+ 58 per cent
Taken into their 40s	+ 144 per cent

The breast cancer rate in the UK is one in eight women. If a woman takes the pill in her forties, as over 10 per cent of the UK population does, the risk is estimated at one in three!

The Women's Health Initiative in the USA was a major study looking into a number of health issues. One part, where 16,000 healthy women aged between 50 and 79 were involved in a major clinical trial, the women using synthetic oestrogen and progesterone mixed HRT pills showed increases in breast cancer of 100 per cent plus increased rates of heart attacks, strokes and blood clots in the lungs. The trial was stopped 5.2 years into the 8 years for this combined pill, but still continued for the oestrogen-only pill where breast cancer increases were only around 27 per cent. (To put this figure in context, the increased risk of cancer, any cancer, attributed to smoking is 25 per cent, according to the late Sir Richard Doll and team in their pioneering work on tobacco). The FDA joined in the warnings insisting that HRT packaging contained a warning. However that warning was for increased risk of heart problems not cancer!

Cancer Research UK found almost the same increases in risk in its '*Million Women*' study – the leading synthetic oestrogen/progesterone brand doubled the risk of cancer, whilst oestrogen-only increases it 26 per cent. Findings also showed that HRT makes 'breast screening' less effective and breast cancer patients who were on HRT are 22 per cent more likely to die from the disease.

None of this is new. *The Boston Nurses Questionnaire Study* results were published almost ten years before, says Sherrill Sellman, an expert in oestrogen. It followed 121,700 women for 18 years. Ten years of oestrogen alone showed the cancer risk rising by a third, whereas the mixed pill doubled risk. The American Cancer Society in a further analysis involving 240,000 post-menopausal women (1995) showed that the risk of fatal ovarian cancer was 40 per cent higher for women using the HRT pill for at least six years and 70 per cent higher after 11 years.

There is also evidence for girls in their formative years. Sellman confirms that the "earlier a girl goes on the pill the greater her eventual risk of contracting breast cancer, the larger her tumours and the worse her eventual prognosis." Sellman adds, "Oestrogen dominance actually accelerates the ageing process, increasing the risk of endometrial cancer and ovarian cancer, blood clots, strokes and high blood pressure."

In 2005 2.2 million women in the UK took HRT; a third over 50 took it, and half will take it at some time in their lives. The NHS dispensed 6 million prescriptions at a cost of £133 million. Bad press did see a fall of users, and a decline in breast cancer rates, but that is long gone.

Dutch doctors writing in the Lancet called on women taking HRT to stop immediately – whereas UK doctors told women to balance risks and benefits! The Head of the German Medical Authorities described HRT as '*The new thalidomide*'.

3. Reduce your calories:

High calorie intake also stimulates oestrogen production. (Fat is, of course, high in calories.) An excess of insulin causes some hormones to be depleted whilst others – and notably oestrogen – are produced in larger quantities. Thus the typical Western eating pattern of two big meals a day leads to insulin, and oestrogen, surges. It is better to cut refined carbohydrates from the diet completely and 'graze', as I said earlier, eating six small meals a day and thus controlling excesses of insulin.

Insulin is primarily produced in response to a diet high in refined carbohydrates and sugars. Insulin prevents high blood sugar levels damaging the brain.

Harvard Medical School calculated that a **5 per cent increase in calorie intake is associated with a 20 per cent increase in oestrogen levels, through the 'insulin link'.**

However, calorie restriction and even fasting are being shown in research to halt cancer progression. Calorie restriction diets, such as those endemic to inhabitants of Okinawa, or wartime diets in Europe see an increase in health and longevity.

4. Want to reduce breast cancer risk? Have another baby!

Another way (obviously unique to women) that oestrogen excesses are made is the modern attitude to babies.

Diet primarily affects women's fertility. Women two hundred years ago were 'productive' normally from 16 to 38 years of age. They also had four to five children and breastfed them for at least a year and even two. Now the average New Yorker can have periods from age 12 to 52 and only one child, which she rarely breastfeeds for more than a few months, if at all. As a result her number of periods has doubled from 200 or so to 400. So, that's twice as many oestrogen surges by the time she reaches 50 as her ancestors were used to. Dr Pollard has shown that women in Mali, West Africa, have an average of 109 periods compared to a typical Western level of 400.

Cancer Research UK has confirmed that having more babies and breastfeeding longer can cut breast cancer rates. (Having another baby is their idea, not mine!) For every extra child there is a 7 per cent reduction; and a 6 per cent reduction for breastfeeding the child to month nine.

The Bush people in Australia or the Kalahari breastfeed their children until they are almost 5 years old in a toxin-free environment. They have no breast cancer.

5. Cut your cows' dairy consumption:

Cows' dairy can dramatically affect your oestrogen levels too:

*   * Its fat content brings with it a variety of toxins including oestrogen and oestrogen mimics as we saw above.
*   * Dairy-dominated diets depress magnesium. Magnesium works a little pump found in the cell wall. The job of this pump is to expel sodium and push in potassium so that the cellular power stations can work properly. Without this action, the havoc caused is very similar to that of oestradiol.
*   * Separate American, Swedish and Japanese research studies show that dairy can negatively affect your

cells. Dairy, especially in the USA where growth hormones are used with cattle, contains Insulin-like Growth Factor (IGF-1), which in the presence of milk protein more easily enters the human blood stream. Normally produced by the pituitary in very small amounts, IGF-1 has been linked to changes in cellular metabolism, malignant cell proliferation and cancer in women and men *(Cancer Prevention Coalition, Chicago and NCI)*.

* There appears to be a fair degree of cross-talk between the two hormones. There is increasing evidence that oestradiol and IGF-1 act through a complex cross-talk mechanism to stimulate cells resulting in breast cancer. "The emerging model of cross-talk suggests that oestradiol regulates the expression of IGF-I and the IGF receptor. The subsequent binding of IGF-I to its receptor initiates an intracellular signal pathway that activates transcription factors, including the oestrogen receptor *(Mary Beth Martin and Adriana Stoica, Journal of Nutrition 2002)*. Put simply, oestradiol helps IGF-1, which in turn reciprocates.

Swedish research announced in 1999, indicated **a direct line link between the level of dairy consumed and a male's risk of prostate and testicular cancers!** The line isn't so accurate for **breast cancer,** but the evidence suggests **the more you consume, the greater your risk of breast cancer.**

A study carried in Cancer Watch on ovarian cancer showed women who consume the equivalent of more than two cups of milk a day have a doubled risk of ovarian cancer.

6. Sodium is a serious endocrine disrupter:

And significantly inhibits the production and the action of certain hormones.

And as we have said, if one hormone goes out they all go out, making your body toxic and cancer more likely. But we all eat too much sodium. Sausages, bacon, crisps, peanuts, fast food, processed foods, dried meats like hams and salami: Do you recognise the diet??

Four slices of white or malted bread, three bags of crisps or three bowls of breakfast cereal each provide 1 gram of sodium! Worse are processed foods, monosodium glutamate and even soy sauce. Some fast food outlets 'healthy' salads contain over 4 gms in one meal!

The average American eats a massive 12 gms per day of sodium, the average Brit about 10 gms. The FSA in the UK has decreed a safe level of 6 gms for adults and 3 gms for children. In the wild thousands of years ago, an animal was unlikely to have eaten any at all. So much so that salt licks needed to be found. In Roman times salt was a form of currency, because of its scarcity. The word sal meaning salt, gave rise to the word 'salarium'. I feel strongly that a level of 1 to 2 gms per day is ample, and this is the figure decreed by the US Institute of Medicine in February 2004.

Meanwhile you should eat more potassium and magnesium.

High potassium and high magnesium foods include pulses, like lentils, chickpeas, broad beans, peas, kidney beans etc, nuts, brown whole rice, bananas, apples, green leafy vegetables, and jacket potatoes.

You should eat five times more potassium a day than sodium to ensure your cells and your hormones stay healthy and balanced.

7. Oestrogen prescriptions:

All the scientific indications are that we all have far, far more oestrogen in our bodies than nature intended. Yet doctors seem to want to give us more of it. For example, HRT is given supposedly because oestrogen levels fall dramatically at the menopause. But since they start in modern women at far higher levels than were present in her ancestors, where is the evidence that they have fallen too low and need supplementing with synthetic oestrogen? Indeed, natural oestrogen levels only fall to about 60 per cent of 'normal' – just enough to prevent ovulation. Whereas progesterone falls completely, with about 3 per cent of original levels being produced by the adrenal glands. In men several studies seem to indicate that our oestrogen pool (of hormones and mimics) simply slowly grows as we age!

a) Osteoporosis?

In the West we have the highest levels of circulating blood calcium and the lowest levels in our bones. Why? Because you need magnesium to get it into the bones and dairy suppresses magnesium. Catch twenty two. Other modern lifestyle factors are also relevant, for example a lack of load-bearing exercise (which is why men are now getting it more frequently) and stress which causes bones to leach calcium. Over use of steroids is another cause, as are excess caffeine and sodium both of which leach calcium from the bones.

Finally, vitamin D (which we largely get from sunshine and a little from fish oils) is low in most of us. The government's and major charity's misguided advice to keep out of the sun has caused a generation of children, men and women to have low levels of vitamin D in their blood streams. Yet vitamin D is essential if you want stronger bones. Vitamin D is essential to a strong immune system. Harvard Medical School recommends 5,000 International Units a day as a supplement if you have cancer. One week of a beach holiday would provide 70,000 IUs. Scientists are still not sure how, but vitamin K (found in greens) is consumed less and less, yet it helps vitamin D work with the immune system and in assimilating calcium into bones.

Women with low levels of vitamin D, magnesium and fish oil compounds in their blood streams develop significantly more breast cancers.

b) Hot flushes and night sweats?
Research shows these can be corrected with natural progesterone just as effectively as synthetic oestrogen.

In fact, all the indicators are that women in the West have much higher levels of oestrogen in their blood streams than women in the East **even after the menopause.** The same applies to men. And cancer rates are far, far lower historically in the East and more primitive countries. Dr Pollard has been taking evidence worldwide and proving exactly this point.

Sadly the reason synthetic oestrogen is recommended like 'sweeties' is that day in, day out usage is big business. Very big business.

On the other hand, natural progesterone can be processed from inexpensive herbs and cannot be patented, so no companies will get rich from it.

8. Direct and Indirect causes of cancer:

Professor Karol Sikora, former head of the World Health Organisation's cancer programme, in his speech 'The future of cancer care', claimed that of the 10 million new cancers worldwide each year, 3 million are due to dietary inadequacies, 3 million due to toxins and pollution, and 1.5 million are due to infection (e.g. viral). He further believes that cancer treatments in the UK pay no attention to these factors – and he is right. But please do not think that the causes of cancer fit neatly into one of these boxes. It simply doesn't work like that.

Cancer is a multi-step process; one report said it took six steps to turn a normal cell into a rogue cell; another, twenty. However, some factors e.g. asbestos or talcum powder may possibly short-circuit all the steps of cancer production. (Talc, asbestos-like in its formula, has been linked to ovarian cancer).

But in most cases, I suspect that the true 'cause' of cancer is indirect. As we said, even a normal healthy individual produces 200–1000 'cancer' cells per day.

But a normal healthy individual has a strong immune system that identifies and neutralises them. So it follows that to avoid cancer, one essential is simply 'Love your immune system'. **American research has shown that people with weak immune systems get more cancers.** Your aim must be to have the strongest possible immune system.

But many chemical products are far more likely to cause indirect effects (like lowering the immune system) than direct effects. I found research from each of the following - the CPC Chicago, Athlone Institute of Technology, Ireland, the NCI in the USA – saying that excess oestrogen and especially pesticides and toxic oestrogen mimics have been clearly shown to weaken the immune system.

At the **icon** offices, our observation is that the great majority of newly diagnosed cancer patients are **nutritionally toxic** (for example, from too much salt, junk food, processed food, lack of vegetables and fruit etc) and/or **nutritionally deficient**. The latter has been borne out by the French Su Vi Max study published in Autumn 2003. 17,000 adults between 35 and 60 years of age were given an anti-oxidant supplement containing beta-carotene, vitamin E, vitamin C, selenium and zinc. In seven years this resulted in a 31 per cent decline in male cancers and, crucially, a 37 per cent decline in cancer mortality for both men and women.

If you have a weak immune system you are more open to attack from a variety of 'predators', for example **yeasts, viruses** or **parasites**. A weakened immune system can allow a virus to take hold. Professor Robert Souhami, Director of Clinical Research for Cancer Research UK, says: "Around 15–20 per cent of all cancers are caused by viruses, so it's vital that we get a better handle on the role of viral infection." For example, some **breast cancer** patients (perhaps only 1–2 per cent) have been found to have the **shingles** virus. About the same proportion of **prostate patients** have been found to have the **herpes** virus.

In fact, these figures could be a vast underestimate. The role of viruses in research was studied until 30 years ago then dropped. Now with better equipment reports from the USA on mouse viruses and breast cancer, or virus studies in Australia, suggest 40 per cent of cancer may be viral.

Cervical cancers have been linked to the Human Papillomavirus; **ovarian** cancer may be triggered sometimes by chlamydia.

CHAPTER 11
ARE THEIR ANY OTHER FOODS WHICH CAN HELP AGAINST OESTROGEN?

1. Controlling the oestrogen pathways: The National Cancer Institute in the USA found in 2003 that obesity is linked to a 40 per cent increase in cancer risk (by comparison, smoking increases it 25 per cent). Other studies suggest obesity is linked to a 60 per cent increased risk of cancer.

A researcher from New York University Steinhardt, assistant Professor Niyati Parekh, set out to look at the underlying cause. *"Obese people are more likely to have (abnormal) insulin levels in their blood," Parekh said. "Insulin is the gatekeeper for glucose entering the cells, so when insulin production is disrupted, higher values of glucose remain in the blood ... And an increase of glucose in the blood creates an environment that is conducive for cancer cells to grow quickly."* Remember, cancer cells need glucose – lots of it. Diabetics (who have poor insulin control) have three times the normal risk of developing cancer.

But it's not just an insulin and glucose effect. Animal fat consumption stimulates oestrogen production. **Research shows a 10 per cent increase in fat consumption increases female oestrogen levels by 20 per cent.** Men who enjoy fried breakfasts have a three-fold increased risk of cancer over those who do not partake. Dr Tessa Pollard of Durham University made the front pages of British newspapers in September 2003, with the headline 'DIET CAUSES BREAST CANCER' and stated that *"we tend to eat a lot of fatty food that increases steroid levels and oestrogen is a steroid"*.

Professor Powles of Parkside Oncology Centre, Wimbledon stated a similar view in **icon** magazine recently. *"I agree with Chris Woollams that there is a good argument in reducing animal fat intake"*, he says adding; *"There is evidence that animal fat increases oestrogen levels and that that could be detrimental. We're trying to reduce oestrogen with a lot of treatments we're doing. Our general advice is to reduce animal fats and take unsaturated fats instead."*

Unsaturated fats would typically include Rainbow Diet fats and oils like extra-Virgin Olive Oil, nut and seed oils like coconut oils and flaxseed oil, and fish oils.

One of the problems with overweight people is that their bodies contain more aromatase which breaks down the fat to yield oestrogen. This is particularly clear in overweight men as they age, where the enzyme can also produce oestrogen at the expense of testosterone.

Zinc, selenium, green tea and citrus isoflavones can reduce aromatase action, and **resveratrol** was shown to have an anti-oestradiol activity in 2006 research from the Hong Kong Medical School.

Resveratrol, **quercitin** and **prunetin** have all shown aromatase blocking actions in research. Resveratrol has also been shown to inhibit fatty acid synthesis.

But there are several pathways for oestrogen metabolism in the body. One, which goes along the C-16 pathway, produces more aggressive oestradiol. The one that goes along the C-2 pathway is much safer. Men and women who metabolise oestrogen along the C-16 pathway, have much higher rates of breast and prostate cancer. The safer C-2 (oestrone) pathway is supported by nutrients such as B vitamins, fish oils, phytoestrogens and I3C/DIM. High carotenoid consumption can also reduce oestrogen development and one research study in Cancer Watch talks of carotenoids preventing breast cancer returning.

Of course oestrogen (and oestrogen mimics) are also one of the main toxins stored in fat. If you carry fat round your stomach, think seriously about your Toxic Waste!!

2. Red Clover and genistein: Hippocrates regularly used the herb red clover, which was studied at The Royal Marsden as a possible oestrogen blocker in breast cancer patients, without reaching a conclusion.

Red clover has a long history of use as a medicinal herb. It is an excellent blood purifier that over time gradually cleanses the bloodstream and corrects deficiencies in the circulatory system. But among classic herbalists, it is probably best known as a herb for treating cancer and is found as a central ingredient in a number of herbal anti-cancer formulas, including the Hoxsey formula, Jason Winter's tea and Essiac tea.

Researchers at the National Cancer Institute have confirmed that there are indeed anti-tumour properties in red clover. One, genistein, has the ability to prevent tumours from developing the blood supplies they need to survive, thus starving them and killing them. Genistein is the same biochemical considered to be the main beneficial ingredient in soya. But red clover has a significant advantage over soya, as it contains about ten times the level found in soya of all four main oestrogen isoflavones, including daidzein and genistein. In addition to isoflavones, red clover contains another class of anti-cancer phytoestrogen compounds called coumestans, for example, biochanin and formononetin. Consuming red clover isoflavones results in higher blood levels of daidzein and genistein, moderate blood levels of biochanin, and low levels of formononetin. Soya consumption does not result in any increase in biochanin or formononetin in the blood. Trinovin from red clover actually contains four isoflavones and may have some effect on prostate cancer in tests reported in *Cancer Epidemiology Biomarkers and Prevention* Vol. 11, December 2002. In a proportion of the sample tested there were clear improvements in the disease.

Professor Trevor Powles' comments about the Royal Marsden study at the time were interesting, with a study looking at prevention over two years on 400 women who didn't have breast cancer and were given genistein. (Genistein is used by some doctors and nutritionists like Professor Lawrence Plaskett, Vice Chairman of The Nutritional Cancer Therapy Trust, in the treatment of hormonally driven cancers.)

"We're just starting to do the analysis now, . . . We're looking at all the potential effects on bone, breasts and

hormone levels with naturally occurring sugars like genistein – from soya and red clover – which are phytoestrogens (naturally occurring oestrogens or anti-oestrogens). If the results are negative, it doesn't mean that red clover doesn't work. We might have got the wrong phytoestrogen mix, or wrong dose, so we will do further trials because I'm sure that there will be natural products that will be very beneficial. I think they will help because in Chinese/Far Eastern diets, where these levels are high, breast cancer incidence is low and the level of osteoporosis is low. So there's something in those diets that's protecting people against both diseases."

3. Medicinal mushrooms and hormonally driven cancers: Medicinal mushrooms contain glycoproteins and polysaccharides, like Beta Glucan polysaccharide. These can only rarely be broken by the body, and 4 Nobel prizes have been won showing how they strengthen the immune system and help cells communicate. They actually help hormones do their job better, they help receptor sites receive their messages, and they help the immune cells see the rogue cells more clearly and differentiate them from healthy cells.

The popular mushrooms on the list are Shiitake, Maitake, Cordyceps, Coriolus, Reishi, Phellinus Linteus and others. Many have hormone normalising characteristics. Researchers at the New York Medical Center led by Dr Sensuke Konno, the head of Urology showed that Maitake mushrooms could shrink a tumour by 70 per cent and in some cases the tumour disappeared. Cancers treated included prostate and bladder. Researchers believed the mushroom had a powerful effect on a cancer-driving enzyme. They also did experiments with the mushrooms and Interferons having similar results *(British Journal of Urology, Dec 2009)*. Research on Reishi has shown it can restrict blood supplies to prostate cancer; a variety of medicinal mushrooms were shown by Perth Medical School to have an effect against breast cancer – eating them two times a day, prevented the cancer returning. Other studies showed a mixture of these mushrooms increased survival times in both prostate and breast cancer patients.

4. Flaxseed: Flaxseed and lignan consumption shows up in the urine. And women with the highest levels in their urine have the lowest levels of breast cancer, a finding shown in studies from America to Japan. Secoisolariciresinol (SDG) is the natural lignan found in flaxseed. Research shows SDG has a direct effect on human oestrogen metabolism and also on its receptor sites on cells. Research in Cancer Watch shows SDG stops the action of oestrogen in stimulating cancer cells.

SDG also increases the production of 'Sex hormone binding globulin'. This binds oestrogen, reduces the free oestrogen in the body, and reduces the stimulatory effect of oestrogen on cell division. In research where animals were given a high fat diet and cancer cells, flaxseed reduced the levels of cancer found when it was also added to the mix. Animals with a highly potent metastatic cancer line had their tumours reduce in size and metastasis almost stop when given high levels of flaxseed.

Two studies with animals given a cancer-inducing chemical for 13 weeks, showed less cancers and smaller tumours if the animals also took SDG, one study reported 46 per cent less cancers if pure SDG was used.

Post-menopausal women given flaxseed supplementation for seven weeks showed increased levels of properly metabolised oestrogen in their urine. Another test on women newly diagnosed with breast cancer showed that factors associated with tumour growth fell 33 per cent in the group taking flaxseed.

Lignans and flaxseed pass through the body in 24 to 48 hours so daily consumption is essential.

5. Polyphenols: Other plant 'ingredients' that have been found to be very protective in hormonally driven cancers are polyphenols. Green Tea contains very potent polyphenols and various studies from Perth University, the Mayo Clinic in the USA and others have shown it can reduce breast, prostate, skin cancer and leukaemia risks and effects.

Dr. Keith Singletary and his team have shown that sulforaphane, found in Brussels sprouts, broccoli and cruciferous vegetables, can inhibit the development of breast cancer by binding to the receptor sites and preventing oestrogens 'locking on'.

6. Sterols: Sterols promote natural progesterone formation in the body and reduce oestrogen production. They also promote testosterone formation. Raw nuts, seeds and olives are good sources, and they also contain natural vitamin E which has anti-oestrogenic activity too.

7. Chlorophyll has powerful anti-oestrogenic benefits. Wheatgrass would be a strong source. And seaweeds and algae are known to reduce oestrogen activity. One bioactive compound of benefit in seaweeds is fucoidan.

CHAPTER 12
HOW DO OESTROGEN LEVELS CHANGE?

1. Doctors measure oestrogen levels by taking blood tests. This is wrong. The only accurate measurement is to take saliva tests. A blood test will not just measure free oestrogen, but also protein-bound (non-bioavailable) oestrogen. Worse, blood tests measure plasma or serum levels but most of the free oestrogen is carried by the red blood cells and escapes measurement. (Cummings et al *NEJM* September 1998).

2. Not only is a blood test of oestrogen inaccurate but the whole idea of measuring oestrogen on its own is absolutely irrelevant. The only relevant measurement of oestrogen is its level relative to progesterone since, in their natural state, they are mutually balancing.

3. For women, conventional medicine will tell you that at menopause your 'symptoms' (hot flushes, osteoporosis, heart attack risk) are brought on by the sudden fall of oestrogen. In fact **this is simply not true**. Your oestrogen level gradually declines over the decade before the menopause.

   Secondly, the implication is that oestrogen levels have suddenly declined to zero. In fact, **oestrone falls** only about 40 per cent, and oestradiol about 60 per cent during this time. So by no means is this decline 'total', or even near total. There easily remains enough 'oestrogen' to keep all bodily functions intact save for egg production and pregnancy.

However, at the same time a hormone (the sex hormone binding protein, SHBC) has grown in volume and this blocks the action of the remaining oestrogen causing some of the post-menopausal symptoms. This blocking hormone can be neutralised by natural progesterone.

4. However progesterone has declined severely in the decade before menopause to almost zero levels. A little – about 3 per cent of original levels – is produced by the adrenal glands.

5. A healthy ratio of progesterone to oestradiol (in accurate saliva tests) is 200:1 to 300:1. However after menopause this ratio is greatly exceeded, especially in the modern era where the oestrogen pool has been increasing. Options are therefore to restore some balance with natural progesterone or restrict oestrogen production. Within oestrogen production, it is important to also avoid the C-16 oestradiol pathway, in favour of the C-2 ostrone alternative. Even in men this is the case, where oestradiol far outweighs progesterone levels after menopause. Only recently has the medical profession even contemplated that men might have a menopause.

6. Synthetic progesterone cannot replicate the effects of natural progesterone in this equation; natural progesterone is a precursor for and regulator of, hormones like oestrogen and testosterone through a natural enzymatic feedback system. Like synthetic oestrogens (xenoestrogens), synthetic progesterone has no influence on this feedback system but does have some serious side effects. For example, it increases the risk of coronary problems while natural progesterone prevents them. Furthermore, synthetic progesterone seems to block many androgen receptors and therefore the action of a number of important hormones.

As Dr Contreras, one of the top integrated cancer doctors in the World and head of The Oasis of Hope Hospital, Mexico said to me, the issue with hormonally driven cancers is simple: "Cut the oestrogen"and this is especially true as you age. This strategy is confirmed by leaders of the orthodox medical world too like Professor Trevor Powles. The female drug Arimidex (or Anastrozole) is aimed at post-menopausal women at risk of breast cancer and works simply by 'cutting these women's high levels of oestrogen'. Anybody who has studied the detailed biochemistry of these hormones knows this to be the true solution. There are a number of ways of doing this as we shall now list.

The science of oestrogen and the balancing natural progesterone is also detailed by experts such as the late Dr John Lee and Sherrill Sellman who have spent long periods of research on the subject. Their conclusions are well documented and clear, with supporting scientific evidence.

CHAPTER 13
THE ANTI- OESTROGEN CHECKLIST

Stop
1. Don't be overweight. Work on getting yourself to an ideal weight.
2. Avoid saturated fats, fried food, trans fats.
3. Avoid cows' dairy
4. Eat less calories than you need.
5. Avoid glucose and refined carbohydrates, biscuits, cakes, chocolate, sticky buns
6. Avoid common salt

Go
1. Take light daily exercise – for a minimum of 30 minutes. Try Yoga, meditation and Tai Chi.
2. Sleep in a darkened room; have a regular bedtime; use shades if you need to; take 3-6 mgs of melatonin 30 minutes before going to bed; or look into Asphalia.
3. Go organic. Avoid pesticides.
4. Drink clean water. Glass bottles of mountain water are best. Or you can fit a proper water filter system
5. Clean up your home; no toxins; no EMFs, fizzy soft drinks etc
6. Go toxin-free in your personal care products (look into companies such as Neways)

7. Talk to an expert about natural progesterone
8. Protect your microbiome
9. Eat 6 small meals a day
10. Eat a Rainbow Diet
    a. Major on colours – carotenoids, like red and yellow peppers; anthocyanins, like dark red plums and beetroot; quercitin, like apples, onions
    b. Major on phytoestrogens – eat broccoli and greens, lignans and pulses
    c. Major on good fats – extra virgin olive oil, nut and seed oils like walnut, coconut, pumpkin and sunflower seeds
    d. Major on whole foods
    e. Use flaxseed on your breakfast
    f. Take fish oils every day, maybe a small 75mg aspirin, and eat garlic and ginger
    g. Go in the sun for one hour every day, or supplement with 5,000 IUs of vitamin D3
    h. Supplement if you need
        i. Indole3carbinol/DIM
        ii. Resveratrol
        iii. Quercitin
        iv. B Complex
        v. Medicinal mushroom extract
        vi. Red clover
        vii. Curcumin

THE HOUR GLASS

When people with cancer ring us up at **icon**, the first question we ask is, "is it hormonally responsive?" Hardly anyone seems to know the answer to this really important question. Go and ask your doctor. If the answer is yes, then there is so much you can do to help yourself. We liken it to an hour glass.

The Top 'Bowl'

Consists of changing your eating habits. Smaller meals, 5–6 times a day, less salt, no refined carbohydrate, no insulin rushes, no sugar, fizzy soft drinks. Clean, oestrogen-free water. Phytoestrogens, pulses, fruits. Roughage, isoflavones and garlic (which both limit cancer spread). And supplements.

The Centre

Go and talk to an integrated doctor about natural progesterone treatment.

The Lower 'Bowl'

Clean up your house; repaint if the paint is over 15 years old; beware chipboard, carpet and ceiling tiles – the glues might be toxic.

Don't put perfumes or perfumed products on your skin, or use talc, or toiletries, cosmetics, creams and toners with toxins in them. (Don't put toxic ingredients near your children.)

Don't breathe toxic gases from bleaches, disinfectants, polishes and cleaners, or petrol fumes. Keep computers and faxes downstairs.

Switch to a supplier of toxin-free products like Neways.

APPENDICES

15 CHEMICALS OF CONCERN IN YOUR PERSONAL CARE PRODUCTS

Is your bathroom cabinet bulging with toxins? Is your make-up or toilet bag a cocktail of chemicals that could do you harm? Yes is probably the answer to both of those questions. The higher up the list of ingredients these 15 come, the greater the concentration. So check your products today, then chuck out and buy safer alternatives.

1. **Formaldehyde** – Combined with water, this toxic gas is used as a disinfectant, fixative, germicide and preservative in deodorants, liquid soaps, nail varnish and shampoos. Also known as formalin, formal and methyl aldehyde, it is a suspected human carcinogen and has caused lung cancer in rats. It can damage DNA, irritate the eyes, upper respiratory tract and mucous membrane, and may cause asthma and headaches. It is banned in Japan and Sweden. Can appear under 50 or so different names in ingredients lists.

2. **Phthalates** – repeatedly hit the headlines for being 'gender benders'. They are a family of industrial 'plasticisers' already banned in the EU from being used in plastic toys, but are still in hairsprays, top-selling perfumes and nail varnishes. You can also ingest them as they leach from PET and soft plastic bottles into your healthy designer water and the kids' fizzy drinks. They can be absorbed through the skin,

inhaled as fumes and ingested from contaminated food or breastfeeding. Animal studies have shown they can damage the liver, kidneys, lungs and reproductive system – especially developing testes.

3. **Parabens** – are listed as alkyl parahydroxy benzoates – butyl/methyl/ethyl/propyl/isobutyl paraben on some toothpastes, moisturisers, deodorants, antiperspirants and even sunscreens. They are used as a preservative, and are probably the 'safest' preservative, although some people feel they act as oestrogen mimics. Recent research suggests that parabens in antiperspirant deodorants might cause breast cancer. However, other research suggests parabens are not absorbed through the intestine, and through the skin it is rapidly degraded, while any reaching the blood is quickly hydrolysed. Research has also brought into question any effect on cell receptor sites but none the less parabens accumulate in breast cells and other cancer tissues. So while the jury is out it is best to avoid products containing parabens for now. The problem for manufacturers is what to use instead of parabens.

4. **Sodium Lauryl Sulphate (SLS)** – is one of the major ingredients in nearly every shampoo, bubble bath, liquid soap etc. Why, when it is a known skin irritant, stops hair growth, can cause cataracts in adults, damage children's eye development and cause urinary tract infection? It's cheap and produces lots of bubbles when mixed with salt. Hardly

compensation! Sodium Laureth Sulphate (SLES) is a slightly less irritating form of SLS, but may cause more drying. Both can lead to potentially carcinogenic cocktails of nitrites and dioxins forming in shampoos and cleansers, by reacting with other ingredients. Most importantly SLS weakens the impermeability of the skin allowing about 40 per cent more toxins across and into the blood stream.

5. **Toluene** – is a common solvent found in nail enamels, hair gels, hair spray, and perfumes. It is a neurotoxin and can damage the liver, disrupt the endocrine system and cause asthma.

6. **Alpha Hydroxy Acid** – Long-term skin damage can result from using products containing AHAs (sometimes listed as triple fruit acids, lactic acid, sugar cane extract or glycolic acid). They exfoliate, not only damaged layers of skin but the skin's protective barrier as well. This can decrease protection from the sun by 30 per cent and increase the absorption of chemical ingredients never meant to get through.

7. **Alcohol** – We're talking about the kind found in ingestible products here, like mouthwash. Children have died from accidentally swallowing too much of it. Mouthwashes with an alcohol content of 25 per cent or more have been linked to an 8-fold increase in mouth, tongue and throat cancer risk.

8. **Propylene Glycol** – is a cosmetic form of mineral oil

(refined crude oil) used in industrial antifreeze. People handling it are warned by the manufacturer to avoid skin contact and wear respirators and rubber gloves etc, and yet this is a major ingredient in most moisturisers, skin creams, baby wipes and sunscreens. Why? It's cheap and gives the 'glide' factor in body lotions – but is in fact robbing lower layers of skin of moisture. Lanolin and collagen also clog pores and cause skin to age faster than if nothing was used.

9. **Talc** – increasingly recognised as carcinogenic, having a similar chemical structure to asbestos, and has been linked to an increased risk of ovarian cancer and general urinary tract disorders. So don't dust it on your baby's, or anyone else's, bottom! And certainly don't breathe it. Some cans have a warning saying 'Don't use near nose or mouth. So what is face powder? And where do you use that?

10. **Xylene** – is listed as xytol or dimethylbenzene on nail varnish bottles. It can damage your liver, is narcotic in high concentrations and causes skin and respiratory tract irritation.

11. **Parfum/perfume** – A typical cosmetic can contain up to 100 chemicals in the perfume alone! 95 per cent of these chemicals are synthetic compounds derived from petroleum – 26 of which are on an EU hit list. Fragrances have been linked to allergies and breathing difficulties and they penetrate the skin. The Swedes have research linking perfumed

products to high levels of DEHP in the body. This is a highly toxic oestrogen mimic.

12. **Diethanolamine** – Also Tri and Mono (DEA, TEA and MEA) are absorbed through the skin where they accumulate in organs. When found in products also containing nitrates, they react and form nitrosamines which are carcinogenic.

13. **Aluminium** – is found in most deodorants, has been linked to Alzheimer's, and is increasingly being linked to cancer.

14. **Triclosan** – sometimes listed as 5-chloro-2 (2,4 dichlorophenoxy)-phenol, is in deodorants, toothpastes, vaginal washes and mouthwashes. Toxic dioxins are produced during its manufacture or incineration. It is stored in breast milk and in fish, and can break down in chlorinated water to create chloroform and other toxins.

15. **Paraphenylenediamine** – or PPD is used in dark hair dyes. Tests on rats have shown that PPD may cause cancer, after long-term use with hydrogen peroxide. It has been implicated in numerous bladder cancer cases in California. The perfect excuse to go blonde?

In the UK, call The Natural Selection Shop on 0203 186 1006 for more information on safe products, or go to www.ournaturalselection.com.

As Safe As Houses

'50 per cent of cancers are your own fault' ran the front page headline in a well known UK daily paper, early in 2008. Apparently, it's your lifestyle - we all eat badly, we smoke and drink too much, we go in the sun and we don't exercise enough. The Government and top cancer charities, in their infinite wisdom, are quite clear: We are all to blame for our own potential demise.

Unfortunately for this theory, I receive all too many letters from people who don't smoke, do watch their weight, joined the gym, took up yoga, and gave up the demon drink............. yet, they still got cancer.

So, pray tell, oh wise ones, what causes the other 50 per cent?

The evidence is there; about 20 per cent are caused by infection - viruses, parasites and bacteria. So now let's ask the question again. What causes the other 30 per cent?

Scientists, experts, toxicologists and the like have researched and concluded. It's just that vested interests play a significant part in the denial game.

A good place to start for research into Environmental toxins would be the 2006 report from the *University of Massachusetts, Lowell*: ***"Environmental and Occupational Causes of Cancer: A Review of Recent Scientific Evidence"***. This starts by referring to the report mentioned above and produced by Sir Richard Doll and Richard Peto who attributed only 2-4 per cent of cancers to environmental and occupational exposure.

The new report concludes that, *"Unfortunately this has determined our thinking ever since. Worse, new evidence shows they are clearly wrong."*

In the 50 page study from Lowell, researchers conclude, *"Many cancer cases and deaths are caused or contributed to by involuntary exposures. These include:* **bladder cancer** *from the primary solvent used in dry cleaning,* **breast cancer** *from endocrine disruptors like bisphenol-A and other plastics components,* **lung cancer** *from residential exposure to radon,* **non-Hodgkin s lymphoma** *from solvent and herbicide exposure, and* **childhood leukemia** *from pesticides The authors further noted that the mortality rate for all cancers combined (excluding non-melanoma skin cancer) is the same today as it was in the 1940s, yet the annual rate of new cases has significantly increased"*.

"Major cancer agencies have largely avoided the urgency of acting on what we know to prevent people from getting cancer in the first place," said researcher Genevieve Howe at Lowell.

So, it's certainly not all your fault. And some pressure groups (the Environmental Working Group), and some companies (Johnson & Johnson) and even the EU, where Euro MPs have voted to kick out 1000 common ingredients from common products, are convinced that common chemicals in everyday use, do pose a serious threat to your health. In 2013 the World Health Organisation added its voice saying endocrine hormone disrupters like BPA, phthalates and parabens should be banned.

But many governments and even major cancer

charities live in denial. It's enough to make you retreat into the safety of your own home and bolt the door. Unfortunately, inside your own home is where your problems really start.

Warning: Your home can seriously damage your health

People love to look in estate agents windows. 4 bedrooms, a downstairs loo, en suite shower, wonderful. However, top of the list should come the most important criterion of all: Location.

If you go to UK cancer charity websites, the causes of lung cancer may include asbestos and smoking. However, American sites will associate as many as a quarter of cases with other factors for example, diesel fumes. Breathing toxic particles from diesel fumes will deliver the toxins to the deepest recesses of your lungs from where they are extremely difficult to remove. Epidemiology studies show the dangers of living near main roads and, especially for children, living near petrol stations.

You may of course head to the hills. However, in certain parts of Britain, notably the West Country, areas of Wales and areas round Manchester and Glasgow, our land is rock-based and contains deposits of uranium. The decomposing uranium gives off radon, a colourless, tasteless, odourless gas which slowly bubbles to the surface through your floors. You could try opening all the doors and windows, but this is not too effective as the radon sticks to dust particles in the localised environment of the house. When you breathe in, these dust particles also go to the deepest recesses of your lungs and the radon decomposes further resulting in carcinogenic activity.

Don t be under any illusions about this. Several big studies in the USA, and the US Surgeon General, have concluded that radon is the second largest cause of lung cancer after cigarette smoking. Indeed, if it combines with cigarette smoking, risks are disproportionately multiplied.

One answer, if you are worried, is to contact the Radiological Protection Board on 0800 614529 or visit www.hpa.org.uk/radiation.

Heading for the open countryside may not be much better. There you must avoid a different hazard: Beware farmers bearing toxic sprays. A farmer can spray a fruit orchard as many as 15 times in a season. Not surprisingly farmers have higher incidences of blood cancers like multiple myeloma. Those who live by the spray...

One lady I know in a beautiful Kent oast house had to shut the windows, even on a hot summer day. She developed breast cancer last year. Pesticides and herbicides have been the subject of important papers in the EU. They have even clearly stated that some are proven to be linked to cancer. However the UK Government left pesticides out of their 2004 White Paper on cancer, complete accident, or ignorance, or vested interests? You choose.

Next, avoid living near power cables or electricity sub-stations. Leukaemia risk is increased. At least UK Government policy is now to stop new house building within 200 yards of power cables (not that we're building many houses anyway at the moment!!)

Finally, avoid being down-wind of a factory, especially chemical factories; steel makers, wood cutters/timber merchants or cement factories have all been linked in the USA to increased risk of blood and kidney cancers.

Other Dangers you can't see

Just in case you didn't find that all scary enough, we now have a new threat to our health growing unchecked by our UK leaders. No, not GM foods. **Electrosmog.** The good news so far is that officially in the UK, you can t have a school in the full beam of a phone mast. Precautionary advice, admittedly; but it's a start. We have to protect our little cherubs at school. Of course you can end up living right next to a mast if your local council says the mobile phone boys can erect one in your street, so they may not be very well protected at night.

Until a few started rebelling in late 2007, councils could not turn down a mast planning application on the grounds of safety just on aesthetics. However, the Government of Taiwan know better. They ordered 1500 phone masts to be pulled down and included in the official statement are the words causes health problems and cancer. In **icon** you may have read the story of breast cancer victim Eileen O'Connor and how she proved the presence of a cancer cluster in her village and had her local mast removed.

It s also precautionary advice in the UK that children

should not use mobile phones for long periods. In Canada, their Government has ruled that children under 8 should only be allowed to use mobile phones for emergencies. In China, the Government there simply refuses to allow the sale of mobile phones as strong as those in Britain. Frying tonight was something that only happened down the fish and chip shop when I was a lad. The EU MPs have passed a resolution urging all member states to kick WiFi out of schools and go back to fixed line, plus restrict mobile phone usage and prepare warning leaflets for parents, kids and teachers. No one seems to know about this at all.

Although you may not have WiFi at home, your neighbours may have it the other side of your shared wall. At my mother's UK house, my computer tells me four nearby homes have WiFi strong enough for me to access. (I'm still trying to work out which one amongst them in quiet leafy Epsom is Sexyboots!). The newest threat seems to be the BT hub, which you don't seem to be able to turn off and it doesn t just give you your personal service but contributes to the national grid of WiFi.

Suffer little Children

So, let's assume we have chosen our location wisely. Now let's make a dash for the front door and hope to escape this toxic outside world.

The dangers can start as soon as you walk through the front gate. Moss killers, weed killers, ant killers, rose sprays: If they are harmful to the genes of plants and aphids why would they not be harmful to your genes?

The link between cancer and pesticide exposure is well documented. In one US study, children under 14, whose gardens have been sprayed with herbicides, have a four times greater incidence of connective tissue tumours; in another, pesticides used to eradicate garden insects are linked with increased levels of brain tumours in children and, in another, with a fourfold increase in childhood leukaemia.

As you may be aware, cancer levels have doubled overall in the UK in the last 30 years. What you may not be aware of is that for certain childrens' cancers they have more than trebled.

Several research studies have shown that our children are more susceptible to toxic poisoning (because their brains, nervous and immune systems are still forming) and are more likely to contain toxins in their blood streams.

For example in 2004/5 the **World Wildlife Fund** turned its focus from pandas to humans and, looking for the presence of 78 of the nastiest toxins in everyday life, found 65 of them in our blood streams. On average we have 27, and the highest was in someone from Glasgow with 49 (no comment is necessary). Worse, in a follow up study on 80 harmful ingredients, children were shown, on average, to contain a whopping 75, while the grandparents only had, on average, 56. Importantly, there was no difference at all found between city and rural dwellers. These are inside your home, wherever you may live.

In children the following chemicals were most commonly found:

1. **Polychlorinated biphenyls** from coolants, flame-retardants and plastics: known to affect nervous system and linked to liver and brain cancers.
2. **Organochlorides** from plant pesticides to mosquito repellents: linked to male genital problems and hormone disruptive, oestrogen mimic effects.
3. **Perfluorinated** chemicals from fast food packaging, non-stick utensils, stain resistant carpets and furniture polishes - linked to bladder cancer.
4. **Phthalate**s from plastics in bottles to childrens toys, and many toiletry bottles - known oestrogen mimics and hormone disrupters.
5. **Polybrominated Diphenyl Ethers** found in flame-retardants in cars, furniture and TVs, and in clothing treatments: cause severe hormone disruption and blood disorders.

Worse, not only is the problem occurring inside the home, it seems to stem from the everyday products we bring into the home.

Take another deeply worrying study: In 2008, the University of Washington *(The Journal of Paediatrics)* studying babies between the ages of 2 and 28 months, has found that 80 per cent have blood streams containing seven or more phthalates. The urine of babies who had been exposed to their parents' perfumed lotions, shampoos or powders had four times the phthalate levels of children who had not been exposed to those products. Children under the age of eight months fared the worst. Phthalates are known to be powerful and cumulative endocrine (hormone) disrupters.

Phthalates typically originate from plasticisers used to soften plastic - for example, to make plastic bottles surrounding shampoos and bubble bath. But they can also be found in plastic toys. California has recently banned the sale of plastic toys for children under the age of three. But yours in Britain can play with these toys or even suck on a plastic dummy or a plastic teething ring.

Research has shown that where plastics had contained hot liquids they denatured and released more phthalates, and continued to do so for ever after even when the liquid was cold; so beware thermos cups, plastic cups and beakers, or babies bottles.

California banned their plastic toys in 2007 not just for phthalate content but also because many contain another hormone disrupter Bisphenol A (BPA). You can get yours from certain white linings in cans; baby can get theirs from a plastic feeding bottle.

Canada has banned BPA, full stop. The French want to in 2014. Why can't we?

Direct and indirect cancer causing toxins

Before we continue, it is probably best to provide a little kiddies guide to toxins and cancer.

There are a number of ways you can develop cancer. Suffice it to say that there are certain toxins (radioactivity would be a good example) that can have a direct effect on your cell, and cause a rogue cell to be produced. They may be external, or internal (for example, the free radicals you produce from everyday living).

You make about 200 or so rogue cells throughout each day, but under normal circumstances your immune system mops them up. However if your immune system is impaired, they stand far more chance of beating the system, and you are then on your way to a cancer. There are many things that can weaken your immune system and are thus indirect causes of cancer. Where Cancer Bodies and Governments get their knickers in a twist is that they seem to only want to look at direct causes. And ones that can't sue them, or ones that don't give them money.

So 25 years ago epidemiology studies linked smoking with increased risk of cancer, and warnings were put on pack labels. Science now has theories about how smoking may have both direct and indirect effects, and we are past the point of legal action by Tobacco Companies. But similar epidemiology studies (for example from the Karolinska Institute in Sweden) show that cows dairy is also linked to increased risk of cancer. But farmers vote for MPs. And there are lots of farmers.

IARC, the International Agency for cancer in Lyon, has declared poor sleeping habits carcinogenic. Research shows that lack of sleep reduces melatonin levels and this is linked (probably via two hormones that melatonin seems to control, IGF-1 and Oestrogen) to increased cancer risk, probably directly and indirectly as melatonin is a powerful antioxidant too.

Yet we know that EMFs reduce melatonin levels similarly.

Some chemicals are directly toxic. Heavy metals like cadmium are linked to kidney cancer; mercury to leukaemia. After World War II the worldwide production of chemicals was 1 million tonnes. Now it approaches 500 million. Some chemical compounds like dioxins are extremely, and directly, toxic. Other chemical compounds like phthalates, parabens and BPA can mimic the action of oestrogen when in the body and have a number of serious and negative effects. They are called xenoestrogens and are endocrine disrupters. The World Health Organisation declared in a 2013 report that they were dangerous and should be kicked out. Oestrogen has been proven since 1994 (by the NCI in the USA) to be a cause of cancer; it fuels the fire.

Of course there are Government Safe Limits on each of these hormone disrupting chemical ingredients. But firstly, new research has recently shown some of these to be set way too high. Secondly, Governments approve chemicals in parts per million or parts per billion, but hormones are so powerful they can work at levels of parts per trillion, a thousand to a hundred thousand times less concentrated. Thirdly, Dr Ana Soto of the Tufts Cancer Centre in the USA has shown that xenoestrogens are cumulative in the body. Individually they may all be below Government safe levels - but cumulatively? The US **Cancer Prevention Coalition** covers research that shows the lifetime safe toxin level is exceeded by the time a baby reaches 18 months.

Key Contaminants

We finally make it to the front door. Here it is a good idea to adopt an oriental custom and leave your outdoor shoes outside. Why bring in the lead still found in traces on our pavements, or the germs, pesticides and herbicides into the house and onto the carpets? Again scientific studies have shown that is exactly what you do! Carpets hold over a hundred times more dust than wood flooring and research shows lead levels in carpet dust exceed those in clean-up levels from toxic factory sites! Think about getting rid of your carpets! If not, vacuum at least twice per week and use a vacuum cleaner with at least a HEPA filter.

Relax in the lounge and take a deep breath at the end of a tiring day. Unfortunately, if the radon doesn't get you the **formaldehyde** might!

A 2006 *Columbia University, UC Davis and Harvard School of Public Health* study of teenage kids in LA and New York armed teenagers with air monitors in their back packs and sent them about their normal daily lives. The top pollutants were not quite as expected. First was Formaldehyde, second was Dichlorobenzene. Both these come from indoor sources. A long way behind, and third, was benzene from vehicle fumes. Researchers equated the danger from the top two as being the equivalent of breathing second hand smoke all day.

Formaldehyde is a class A carcinogen (the worst sort) and may be present from a number of sources; for example, the manufacture of cheaper pressed woods (plywood and chipboards), and from some fixatives for carpets and tiles. It is used to stiffen many fabrics like new clothing or upholstery and carpets. It certainly causes respiratory and eye problems and there are several research studies from 2004 and 2005 covered in **icon** linking it to cancers such as lung cancer and leukaemia. The FDA in America supports this concern. Formaldehyde is also contained in many cosmetic and skin and personal care products like nail polishes and shampoos. It is found in household cleaning products, mould and mildew cleaners and even in furniture and contraceptives. Formaldehyde has over 50 different synonyms used by manufacturers to hide its presence; for example methyl aldehyde. It has been banned in Sweden and Japan. Why not in the UK?

So read labels and avoid products containing it; wash all new clothing before wearing it and leave newly carpeted and curtained rooms a week or two with the windows open before you or your children sleep there. Always use 100 per cent cotton sheets and wash them before use.

Dichlorobenzene (1.4-dichlorobenzene) came second in the study and is used in solid deodorisers and mothballs. "Some households had very, very high concentrations and others didnt have much at all", said the lead researcher, who suspects that toilet deodorisers were to blame(!!) Dichlorobenzene is produced from any of these fake, nice smells in the household.

Of course, you have given up **smoking**. But have all those around you? Certainly there is compelling evidence to ask visitors and guests not to smoke in your home. Never allow anyone to smoke in your house.

Research from Cancer Research UK has concluded that the harm from passive smoking is much worse than originally thought. Females are particularly vulnerable, as the risks of smoking link to specific factors in the airways. These factors are produced by the X chromosome. (In our DNA each of us has two chromosomes. Women have two X chromosomes and men have an X and a Y. Thus women produce twice as many X related airway factors).

Lead is another toxin that can enter through those open windows, although less and less as lead-free petrol is widely used now. However, the soil alongside major roads has been found to still be contaminated. Although it has not been proven to be carcinogenic it is extremely toxic to the nervous system, kidneys, blood system and cell reproduction. Lead is still found in paints made before 1980. Maybe its time to brighten up your house. And it is even still found in factories and in tap water.

Tap Water

Many people will shop organically, cut dairy and red meat consumption, eat more vegetables and chant the mantra, You are what you eat, before settling down to a nice cup of tea in front of the TV. There is a weird irony about water in the home. Young lycra-clad women on running machines have their plastic bottled mineral water about them at all times. A symbol of health, indeed fashion. Then they cook in tap water, or eat out in restaurants that do the same.

Tap water has been covered elsewhere in **icon**, and is also the subject of an extensive chapter in our book ***The Rainbow Diet and how it can help you beat cancer.***

Tap water contains chlorine which reacts with organic materials to form highly carcinogenic trihalomethanes. Harvard and other US Health centres have been very active on these chemicals, which are dangerous.

Tap water may contain fluoride. Even the FDA has now confirmed that this is a carcinogen. There are extensive research studies showing that it causes neurological problems and even brain damage especially in the foetus and children. Pregnant women are warned about intake of fluoride. So what should pregnant women do, Mr Prime Minister, if you force through laws to fluoridate all water supplies? Move home while pregnant?

Apart from lead, water can also contain heavy metals like aluminium. Recycled water in major cities can also contain oestrogen and drug levels you most definitely do not need, thanks to HRT, contraceptive pill and drug takers urine.

Increasingly, some tap waters contain chlorine-resistant microscopic parasites.

The safest solution is to drink glass bottled water from pure mountain sources. (Frankly, you cannot be sure that your plastic bottled water is not leaching oestrogen like phthalates into your pure mountain water, so be careful).

Another option is to use a Reverse Osmosis (RO)

Water Filter you can use RO water to wash utensils or to cook. You can of course drink RO water it is commonly drunk in the Far East but normal systems remove almost everything including the minerals and this makes it more acidic. Look for new RO systems that replace the lost minerals and so return the water to its correct state.

Pet Theories

Then you stroke the cat and pat the dog; dog collars and flea collars may keep the pests away from your house, but they too have been directly linked with increased levels of cancer, especially in children. Many have now removed the chemicals of concern. Pet sprays and pet shampoos historically contained pesticides (some have now moved to cut out the worst). Don't laugh, but you can always try feeding your cat garlic and brewers yeast instead? Or try rubbing the fur with clove or eucalyptus oil. The bugs will move on quickly!

To reduce the garden bugs, look for more organic approaches: Vinegar pots kill slugs; good old fashioned fly paper still works, French marigolds keep the aphids off garden vegetables, and chickens eat the moth bugs that descend from the apple trees in winter. Our Grandparent-food growers all knew this.

Don't clean your home!

Ladies - it's official. You mustn't keep your homes so clean.

• The homes of housewives staying at home contain

40 per cent more toxins than those of their sisters who go out to work all day.

• Another study showed that the air in Times Square was 16 times cleaner than inside supposedly clean American homes.

• The American EPA statistics show that women working at home have a 55 per cent increased risk of cancer over those who work away from home!

Most of the harm comes from Volatile Organic Carbons (VOCs). VOCs comprise hundreds, even thousands of man-made and even natural carbon-based agents. Again some of these are known to be direct chemical toxins; while others are indirect immune system weakeners and/or hormone disrupters. We listed earlier in the section on polluted children.

Research carried in icon showed that VOCs can accumulate in certain parts of the body like your lungs, especially at the junctions, and can reach 400 times their original concentrations. Could this be one missing link in the recent Canadian finding that one third of new lung cancer victims have never been near cigarette smoke, even passively, and the incidence of the disease is rising particularly in younger women?

Toluene, xylene, trichloroethylene and l-trichloro-ethane comprise the majority of the solvent market. VOCs are ideal solvents and are also found in pesticides, disinfectants and household cleaners. If you walk down the cleaner aisle of your grocery store you can smell them in the air. The gases can pass through plastic containers; you absorb them by breathing, ingestion or, like the babies in the earlier Washington University study, through absorption via the skin. VOCs have been placed third by the American Environmental Protection Agency, after cigarette smoke and radon, as indoor carcinogens.

VOCs are also found in paints, varnishes, glue for ceiling and carpet tiles, dyes, cleaning products, inks, perfumes, polish removers and more.

We have talked about formaldehyde, but other harmful and common substances include:

- **Phenols:** found in disinfectants, air fresheners, furniture polishes and paint removers. But also in fragrances, nail polish, lip balm, antiseptics, lipstick, mouthwash and other personal care products.
- **Creosol:** found in numerous products from paint removers and disinfectants to personal care products.
- **Benzene and nitrobenzene;** these cross cell walls, damage immune systems and are known carcinogens. Again found in a variety of products from furniture polish to personal care products.
- **Ammonia:** found in cleaners, furniture polish and fabric softeners, but also antiperspirants disinfectants, beauty products, personal care and even baby products!

Lip Service

Never mind the lounge! Worse is to come in your bedroom and bathroom.

In 2006/7 Euro MPs were asked to vote on the

REACH project. This detailed that a number of every day ingredients used in your home contained suspected dangerous chemical ingredients. It wanted those ingredients sidelined, to be replaced by safer alternatives.

The problem is that the makers of household, cosmetic and toiletry products by and large police the safety of their own products. And if their ingredients are not all inert, sadly our Government and leading cancer charities appear to be.

Furthermore, our Governments adopt conflicting standards. A mineral supplement to be taken orally is illegal until you can prove it safe and of benefit. However, the same mineral ingredient in a lotion for your skin that will still reach your blood stream is deemed perfectly safe until you or I prove otherwise.

Quite properly Euro MPs decided certain ingredients should definitely be sidelined. The REACH bill was passed. However that is not quite how Brussels works. Nothing is ever that simple. First the Commissioners have to approve it. However, they were extensively lobbied and decided that the EMPs should reconsider their decision. Result: Mess. (REACH will take perhaps 15 years to implement).

In the USA legislature, 64 bills to ban potentially harmful chemical ingredients have all failed. But the Consumer Groups are winning the day (like the Environmental Working Group). As Johnson and Johnson showed everybody it was possible to come clean in August 2012 when it pledged to eliminate formaldehyde, parabens, triclosan and phthalates from all baby products. For adult products, it has removed triclosan and phthalates, but will keep using three parabens, and use formaldehyde in exceptional cases where other preservatives wouldn t work, according to the company's new policy.

Some MPs jump up and down, write articles and make speeches. But we still have toxic ingredients all around us in the UK. And in a number of cases, the companies bringing these potentially harmful ingredients to our supermarket shelves are the very same ones funding some of our leading universities, professors, charities and their cancer drug research.

That s how to make real profits: Be a part of the problem, and a part of the solution.

And so to bed

Finally, comes the really dangerous bit. It's late, cold and the heating kicks in. Downstairs the gas boiler in the kitchen burns away. You may even have cooked with gas. Whilst old appliances, and especially those with a pilot light, are a significant problem, all gas appliances can cause an increase in nitrogen dioxide levels in the home. It hasn t been proven as carcinogenic to humans, just to animals, although it is known to significantly impair the immune system and have links to arthritis.

You must vent your kitchen to the outside fully and ideally have the gas boiler in a room completely outside the house. Otherwise, the by-products of combustion like nitrogen dioxide will rise through your home, ending up in your bedroom and they can exceed maximum limits set for the gas in polluted city centres!

Still not tired, you pop into your office and flick on the computer; you have a fax to read too. VOCs (including benzene) evaporate from the computer circuitry, laser printers and fax machines in operation. Keep all these machines well away from bedrooms and in rooms which are well ventilated at all times. Don t let your children play computer games upstairs.

And so to bed. You switch on the TV but there s nothing good on, so off it goes and you get into bed, turning the lights off either side of the bed. Ah, a nice, warm, bed; at least the electric blanket works.

Have you considered that the cosy glow you feel may be in part due to the surrounding magnetic radiation? From the TV (turned off, or on standby), the electrical fields generated by the bedside electricity and the electric blanket.

At least the sheets and pillows cases are cotton, now washed in carcinogen-free products, the pillows filled with natural duck feathers not formaldehyde-leaching foamy, plastic stuff.

Sleep deeply in complete darkness and produce that wonderful melatonin. You may need it you make less as you age. I know two UK breast cancer Professors who take it as a supplement every night 1 hour before bed. Unfortunately, whilst Americans can buy this openly in their supermarket that is one thing we actually have managed to ban in the UK and Europe!

CANCERactive

CANCERactive is a UK Registered Charity No. 1102413. Its aims, as agreed with the Charities Commission, are 'to inform and support' cancer patients and to provide 'research' into treatments.

CANCERactive Mission:
The aim of the charity is to provide information, not just on orthodox cancer treatments but on complementary and new, alternative therapies allowing people to make more informed personal choices and so increase their personal odds of survival.

The Trustees of the charity have found that the aim of conducting original research requires funding out of keeping with the funds raised. However, much quality research is available around the world and is not fully communicated to cancer patients. We will fulfil our mission in the 'research' area by providing information on other people's research.

CANCERactive provides the information in a number of ways:

1. A 3400 page website

2. A unique, free magazine called Integrated Cancer and Oncology News (**icon**) available in 600

hospitals, cancer clinics and health centres in libraries.

3. Downloadable prevention leaflets
4. Catherine Corners in Chichester, the Wirral, Hull and Kenilworth.
5. A series of books compiled by Chris Woollams

Readers should note that:
1. All books are compiled and written for CANCERactive by Chris Woollams from information on the website and contained in the research centre Cancer Watch.

2. Neither CANCERactive nor Chris Woollams takes any money from the origination, sale or royalty of these books which are purely designed to provide patient information in line with our agreed Charity Commission remit. Indeed Chris provides all his services to the charity without any remuneration, and we thank him profusely.

Other books include:
The Tree of Life (now *The Rainbow Diet and how it can help you beat cancer*)
Everything you need to know to help you beat cancer
Cancer - your first 15 steps
Oestrogen - the killer in our midst
Conventional Cancer Cures - what's the alternative
The Secret Source of Your Good Health

CANCERactive has neither distribution facilities, nor a sales operation. The Trustees of CANCERactive have appointed Health Issues Ltd (www.ournaturalselection.com) as the sole distributor for all CANCERactive published books and **icon** magazine in the world.

CANCERactive: www.canceractive.com
Tel: +44 (0)300 365 3015

Health Issues: www.ournaturalselection.com